Tell Me What to Eat If I Have Diabetes

Nutrition You Can Live With

by

Elaine Magee, MPH, RD

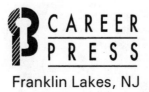

CAREER PRESS

Franklin Lakes, NJ

Author's note: Chapter 1 was reviewed Joseph Barrera, MD, Medical Director of Alta Bates Diabetes Program, Berkeley, CA. Professional experiences were shared by Dorothea Michalik, RD, CDE with Alta Bates Diabetes Program, Berkeley, CA, and Kaiser Permanente Northern California—Faculty for Diabetes Care Management Training.

TELL ME WHAT TO EAT IF I HAVE DIABETES
Cover design by Lu Rossman
Printed in the U.S.A. by Book-mart Press

To order this title, please call toll-free 1-800-CAREER-1 (NJ and Canada: 201-848-0310) to order using VISA or Master Card, or for further information on books from Career Press.

The Career Press, Inc., 3 Tice Road, PO Box 687,
Franklin Lakes, NJ 07417

Library of Congress Cataloging-in-Publication Data

Magee, Elaine.
    Tell me what to eat if I have diabetes : nutrition you can live with / by Elaine Magee.
        p.   cm.
    Includes index.
    ISBN 1-56414-426-7 (paper)
        1. Non-insulin-dependent diabetes—Diet therapy.   I. Title.
    II. Title: Diabetes.   III. Series.
    RC662.18.M34   1999
    616.4'620654—dc21   99-38601

Table of Contents

Introduction

It would make the job of writing this book so much easier if diabetes were a simple disease with a cut-and-dry treatment. But diabetes is a chameleon, manifesting itself differently in different people and sometimes even changing throughout its course within the same person. No one dietary approach, no one medication, works with all diabetics.

What I can offer you in this book is an arsenal of dietary approaches. I can tell you what is working for some people with diabetes and what seems to work for others. Whether or not it helps you and your blood sugars will be up to you to discover. What I won't do in this book is lecture you or tell you diabetes horror stories. You have already heard plenty of those, I'm sure. What you do need is a good friend, well versed in nutrition, who will help you make sense of the situation at hand. I'm going to be that friend. Hopefully, as you read this book, you will feel as though I am holding your hand, walking you through the steps. Together we will find an eating plan that you can not only live with, but love.

The best gift I can give you is to help you approach life as if you don't have diabetes—for many this includes eating foods you love and enjoy. This book will get you closer to that goal. That is my promise.

Chapter 1

The Who, What, Where, Why, and How of Type II Diabetes

D iabetes is reaching epidemic proportions. Roughly 18 million Americans already have this disease and many more will get it in the coming years as baby boomers age and if the rise in adult and child obesity continues. Experts say that about eight to nine million Americans are walking around not knowing they even have diabetes. Often they don't find out until fairly severe damage has been done to their bodies. What kind of damage? Diabetes is the leading cause of blindness, kidney failure, and leg amputations. In fact, it is the third leading cause of death in the United States (depending on whether you include the people with diabetes who die from related cardiovascular disease).

Once you have diabetes, your risk for heart disease can be four times greater. So telling you what to eat for Type II diabetes also has to include telling you what to eat to reduce your risk of heart disease. In fact, the type of food/meal choices that work best for diabetics (lower sugar, lower sodium, high fiber, fruits, and vegetables, with sources of monounsaturated fats and omega-3 fatty acids) is great for someone *without* diabetes. The only difference is that people *with* diabetes need to carefully control and monitor their blood sugar and therefore sometimes need to keep count of carbohydrate, fiber, and fat grams throughout the day.

The bottom line then for most people with Type II diabetes is eating **good food** at **good times** in **good portions.** That's what the rest of this book is all about.

Q **Who is at risk for Type II diabetes?**
   • People age 45 and older.
   • People with a family history of diabetes.
• People who are overweight.
• People who do not exercise regularly.
• Certain racial and ethnic groups (African-Americans, Hispanic-Americans, Asian-Americans, Pacific Islanders, and American Indians).
• Women who have had gestational diabetes or who have had a baby weighing 9 pounds or more at birth.

Q **What exactly does insulin normally do in the body when the body isn't resistant?**
Insulin is a hormone normally produced as needed by the pancreas that converts sugar, starches, and other foods into energy. One of its major jobs is getting glucose (energy) into various body cells. When blood glucose levels rise, the pancreas makes more insulin and releases it into the bloodstream. The insulin then causes body cells to remove the excess glucose that is circulating in the blood. In the liver and skeletal muscle cells, the insulin encourages the production of glycogen (the storage form of glucose). In the liver and fat cells, insulin encourages

fat production (stored energy). At the same time insulin discourages the breakdown of body fat for energy (lipolysis), causing the body to rely more heavily on the recently ingested carbohydrate for current energy needs.

What is Type II diabetes?

Type II diabetes is a metabolic disorder resulting from the body's inability to make or properly use insulin. It occurs when the body produces plenty of insulin, but the insulin cannot do its job. For some reason, the cells in the body have become resistant to insulin. In most cases being overweight or obese for a period of time can bring on insulin resistance. But there are people who are obese for many years who never develop diabetes. So, scientists suspect that some people have a genetic predisposition (their particular family genes make them more likely to develop Type II diabetes under certain conditions such as with aging, weight gain, or an inactive lifestyle).

Ninety to 95 percent of people with diabetes have Type II. About 5 to 10 percent have Type I (usually diagnosed among children or in young adults, and usually not associated with obesity).

What are the warning signs of Type II?

Often people with Type II don't have obvious signs. But they could also have any of the following traditional Type I symptoms:

* Frequent infections.
* Blurred vision.
* Cuts and bruises that are slow to heal.
* Tingling/numbness in hands or feet.
* Unusual thirst.

- Frequent urination.
- Extreme hunger.
- Unusual weight loss.
- Extreme fatigue.
- Irritability.

Q **Why do people get Type II diabetes?**
Not all persons with Type II diabetes are created equal. It acts differently in each person. But most people with Type II diabetes start with the potential to develop the disease (genetic predisposition) based on family history or ethnicity, that eventually becomes manifest through environmental factors such as aging, weight gain, or a sedentary lifestyle.

Q **How will this book help?**
I know it takes some time to accept that you now have diabetes. This may take a few months or a few years, depending on the person. A good friend of mine was in what you could call "diabetic denial" for about two years—not exercising, not really paying attention to her blood glucose, or what she ate. I wrote another book called *The Good New Eating Plan for Type II Diabetes,* and she was one of the first people to whom I gave a copy. Every time I would see her, I would ask if she had read it. She would always have an excuse.

Finally one day she said, "I guess I better start acting like a diabetic." Almost overnight she started monitoring her blood glucose, counting carbohydrates, fat, fiber, and working some exercise into her busy work week. She feels much better now. Guess what? She had finally read the book.

If you are reading this book right now, chances are you are there. You have accepted that this is now a part of your life. You want to make it work for you. You want to manage your blood glucose, reduce your risk of heart disease, and just plain feel better. Then and only then can this book help.

 How can I manage my diabetes?
Many diabetes specialists believe there are three keys to diabetes management success:

1. Monitoring blood glucose levels

You need to monitor your blood glucose because that's how you know right away if you are keeping your blood glucose near normal. And you need to keep your blood glucose near normal if you want to protect your body from developing diabetic complications further down the line. If your health-care team knows how your blood sugar is being affected from day to day, they can help fine-tune your medications, your eating plan, and your exercise routine.

Measuring your blood glucose will tell you rather quickly whether your treatments (diet, exercise, and pharmacological) are working for you. Make sure someone on your health-care team clearly demonstrates how to measure your glucose and how to record it so it can be referred to easily at follow-up visits.

This is very important to the management of diabetes. Next to the discovery of insulin, the ability to monitor blood sugars has been the biggest breakthrough in the treatment of this disease.

2. Exercising regularly

Exercise can actually help control blood glucose levels. Exercise depresses insulin production and also prompts skeletal muscle cells to take in more glucose from the bloodstream. With more glucose in your muscle cells, you can produce more energy so that your muscles can continue to work.

Besides helping to control blood glucose levels, exercise improves the cardiovascular system (thus reducing the risk of heart disease), and it also encourages weight loss, which can have big benefits for people with diabetes.

3. Following a personalized eating plan

Follow a plan that helps keep your blood glucose levels normal, and helps protect against heart disease and weight gain without making you feel deprived. This is the key that this book will give you the most help with.

This book, though, is not about telling you the one and only way to eat—no one diet is best for all people with diabetes. Every person has different risk factors (obesity, hypertension, high triglycerides, kidney dialysis, etc.) that need to be considered. I will tell you generally which foods or meals will be more likely to cause higher blood sugars and will recommend a more moderate carbohydrate and fat eating plan. But when it comes right down to it, every person is affected by the same food or meal a little differently. Chalk it up to unexplained individual differences.

Q **Where can I go for more information?**
- To find a Certified Diabetes Educator in your area (many provide individual consultations and some offer classes for diabetics), contact The American Association of Certified Diabetes Educators toll-free at 800-832-6874.
- For a list of registered dietitians with expertise in diabetes (RD, CDE) in your area, contact The American Dietetic Association's National Center for Nutrition and Dietetics at (800-366-1655) or visit its Web site www.eatright.org and click on "Find a Dietitian."
- The American Diabetes Association maintains a hotline at 800-DIABETES (342-2383), and information on types

of diabetes is available by mail, fax and from staff members. The Association's Web site is www.diabetes.org.

Hopefully your local diabetes center or clinic has a referral sheet available, filled with local numbers for everything from diabetes support groups and counselors to dietitians, diabetes educators, fitness clubs, and personal trainers. If it doesn't, find someone who does. Many hospitals have diabetes support groups and that is a great starting place.

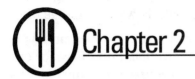 <u>Chapter 2</u>

Top 7 Profiles of Type II Diabetics

I know you feel like you have been wearing the label "Type II diabetes" lately and that health professionals and other people like to lump all Type II's together. The truth is that people with Type II diabetes come in different shapes and sizes and with different health risks and medical problems. Your health risks and medical problems, in addition to having Type II diabetes, also define what needs to be done food-wise to help you feel better and live longer. It is important we get these other issues on the table so that you can get a better idea of what your personal diet/food priorities are and how your Type II diabetes might differ from others.

There are certain trends that stand out in people with Type II diabetes. I've attempted to talk about many of these trends in this chapter. Maybe you will find yourself described in one or more of the following profiles.

1. Waiting to lose weight

Let me first say, you are not alone. I have spent most of my adult life waiting to lose weight. I understand how difficult it is. I know that often thin people actually eat more and exercise less than not-so-thin people (but whose counting?). I know what it is like to eat healthy, exercise every day, and still not lose weight. I have even been told I am too fat to talk about eating healthful on television. But I am the most common size in America—I am a size 14.

One-third of Americans are considered "overweight." But what shocked me was that survey data (National Center for Health Statistics) in 1988-1991 showed a dramatic increase of about 8 pounds in body weight of U.S. adults since the last survey was conducted (1976-1980). It didn't matter which gender, age, or cultural group you looked at—weight gain still followed.

How can this be? Jenny Craig, Weight Watchers, Slim Fast, and other billion dollar dieting giants have been waging war against weight gain for decades now! Never before have more reduced fat foods been available. Getting back to the basics of weight control sheds some light on this rather sore subject.

As you've probably heard, one of the first questions related to weight control is: Do the "calories in" equal the "calories out"? That's because the net effect of excess calories (more than our current body needs), even in the form of carbohydrates or protein, is going to increase the amount of fat put into storage (body fat). We know that most Americans haven't exactly been increasing their "calories out" side of the equation. Due to a combination of modern life factors (television, long commutes, computers, etc.), Americans have become more sedentary.

What about the "calories in" portion? True, the average person ate less fat as a percentage of total calories during the survey period (from 36 to 34 percent)—but the amount of total daily calories went up an average of 231 calories compared to 1976-1980. Aaah...now we're getting to the real million-dollar question: Why would Americans suddenly increase their total daily calories at a time when the country has never been more obsessed with dieting and more concerned about healthy eating?

Ironically, some researchers think it is exactly this overemphasis on fat-free foods that has contributed to the rampant weight gain. Perhaps this wave has fed the belief that if a food has little or no fat, you can have as much as you want without gaining weight. Perhaps when people eat mediocre fat-free foods, it leaves them feeling unsatisfied, so they eat more of the fat-free products, or end up eating something else in hopes of satisfying their hunger or food craving. Maybe since a large chunk of the American population is actively dieting at any one time, they continue to ride the unfortunate weight roller coaster of strict dieting and obsession: deprivation, binging and guilt, strict dieting and obsession, over and over again. Studies show that when people diet, the vast majority of them eventually gain the weight back—and then some. Maybe some of these 8 pounds are the "and then some" from a country that chronically diets.

So what are we going to do about it?

- *Stop dieting*! We know it doesn't work. We know it actually works against you.

- *Eat when you are hungry and stop when you are comfortable*. When we "diet" we force ourselves *not* to listen to our natural hunger cues. When we do this, we also tend *not* to listen to our "comfortable" cues and overeat at times. In order to stop overeating, we need to stop dieting and start listening to when our body truly is hungry and truly is comfortable.

- *Start exercising*! Exercising helps your body in so many ways. It is one of the fastest ways to increase your "calories out" side of the equation. (See Step #10 in Chapter 4 for information about how to exercise if you don't like to exercise.)

- *Start counting* carbohydrates, fats, and fiber as often as you can to gain close control of your blood sugars. I know counting is a big pain, but you don't have to do it all the time for the rest of your life. You might start counting your carbs, fat, and fiber every day until your blood sugars are under control. Then you can do "check in" counting— every week or so or every month if your blood sugars are staying within normal limits.

Logging in what you eat and how you exercise will also help you and your dietitian or Certified Diabetes Educator better understand what small changes might take place to encourage weight loss. Granted, all of the above are easier said than done.

2. I have couch potato-itis

If the first thing doctors told you to do (after being diagnosed with Type II diabetes) was "lose weight," then the second thing they probably told you was to "start exercising." The bottom line is that physical activity can make the difference between losing weight and not losing weight, blood sugar control and out of control blood sugars, going on insulin and not having to go on insulin, taking a high dose of insulin and taking a lower dose of insulin. Regular exercise has been shown to lower high triglycerides levels in the blood and lower high blood pressure after only 10 weeks. The risk of heart attack also decreases with regular exercise.

Exercise does a lot more than reduce risk factors; it has psychological benefits too. It just plain makes you feel better. It tends to encourage better sleep; it gives you more energy throughout the day. It helps you feel better about your body even if pounds haven't been lost, and it helps reduce depression and stress.

I can go over and over all the various and sundry benefits (immediate and down the road) from exercise and physical activity, and I can even hold your hand and follow you around for a month helping you get in the habit of exercising. But sooner or later it is all going to come back to one person—you. Ultimately you have to take responsibility for yourself.

The first step is to commit to trying "exercise" for one month, remembering to start slowly. To see major benefits in your blood sugar control, exercising five to six times a week (even if it is just for 15 minutes each time) is helpful. At the end of one month you should hopefully have experienced many of the psychological and physiological benefits of exercise and you will be adequately "hooked." So let's look at how to get started:

- Visit your doctor and make sure you can proceed with your plans to start exercising.
- Don't make it a big weight loss contest—focus on health and gaining better control of your blood sugar.
- It has to be fun or you are definitely not going to stick with it.
- Next, find out what your exercise preferences/needs are and try to consider them when making your exercise plans.

- Do you like exercising outdoors or indoors?
- Do you like to exercise alone, with a partner, or with a group?
- Do you like the gym atmosphere?
- What time of day would you be most likely to stick to exercising?
- Do you have any physical limitations that need to be considered? If you have joint limitations, for example, water aerobics or swimming can actually be a great starting place.
- What do you like to do? Even if your answer is watching television or talking, they can be worked into your exercise program. If you like to talk, walking with a partner might be the ticket. If you like to watch television, then home exercise equipment that you can use in the comfort of your family room or bedroom might be your most practical option.

Every little bit helps

Even if you can't imagine exercising 30 minutes or more in one sitting, split it up into three 10-minute mini-workouts. Ten minutes of activity here and there does add up to health benefits for your body. Any way that you can increase your activity throughout your day will help your cause.

Home exercise equipment

Stationary and recumbent (back supporting) bicycles are very successful with former couch potatoes. You can literally go from the couch to the bicycle. Position a fan in front of the bicycle if you like. There are a few things to consider when picking out an exercise bike:

- Make sure the seat is adjusted correctly.

- Make sure the seat is wide and comfortable.

- If you opt for a stationary bike, consider the type where the fly wheel gives you a breeze (helping cool you off) and the handles move because this prevents leaning.

Many people make the mistake of buying inexpensive exercise equipment. I know this is tempting. To get the well-made equipment, the kind that will last a lifetime, it will run you around $800 (give or take a couple hundred). This is shocking, I know. But if you buy the cheaper stuff, that creaks when you use it, it will inevitably break or you will tire of it quickly because it isn't as comfortable to use. Isn't buying one well-made piece of equipment better than buying three cheaper pieces that you will stop using after a few months? Many stores offer payment plans of $20 or $30 a month. There are also places that sell used exercise equipment, which can shave quite a bit off the price.

Another home exercise no-no is: Don't buy exercise equipment through catalogs or television infomercials. You want to try it out before you buy it. Literally get your sweats on and go to the store. Tell the salesperson you want to try it out for 20 or 30 minutes. Only then will you be able to tell whether you can comfortably exercise on it for at least 30 minutes at home.

If you want to research the better designed pieces of exercise equipment, look up *Consumer Reports* at your local library. This magazine rates exercise equipment every year. But remember the only way to know for sure how you like it is to just get on and try it.

Exercise videos

I picture exercise videos sitting week after week on a shelf somewhere. But then again, I'm not an exercise video person. I can buy them all right; I just don't ever get the chance to stand in front of my television and watch them. I'd rather be walking outside or watching a movie or television show while I ride my bike. Obviously, some people actually use their exercise videos. In fact, they might even find them motivating. Probably one of the most motivating for larger-sized exercisers are the Richard Simmons tapes which use larger-sized exercisers in the video itself.

You can use videos as a discreet way to try something new (like step classes or kick boxing) in the privacy of your own home. You don't have to worry about what you look like in those jogging shorts or if you will stumble off your "step" in step class because you are the only one there.

If this appeals to you, send for this free catalog, "Complete Guide To Exercise Videos" by Collage (800-433-6769). This catalog lists the tapes by category and tells you exactly what to expect with every video—the type of music, the length, the exercise level, the components of the workout, etc. They offer something for just about everyone— exercise to gospel music, country western dance workouts, and even a hot dance workout video by Paula Abdul.

3. Hyper about hypertension

At least one in every four American adults has it and about 60 percent of people with Type II diabetes have it. The cause is basically unknown. If left untreated it can kill you suddenly, without warning. What is this silent killer? It's hypertension (or high blood pressure). If you have hypertension, chances are you are taking some medication to help control your blood pressure and you might have been told to change your diet in a few different ways.

If you have hypertension *and* diabetes, you probably feel like you are taking an entire handful of medications every day to keep your blood sugar and your blood pressure in check. But if you are able to improve your blood sugar and blood pressure by eating wisely, you may be able to reduce the dosages for some of those medications (and maybe even eliminate one or two of them).

Improving your blood pressure, though, isn't going to make you feel "better," like improving your blood sugar does. You will just have to take my word for it. It's a very good thing—a life saving measure. Both of my parents-in-law died, unexpectedly, in their 50s due to uncontrolled high blood pressure. Two of their children are already on high blood pressure medications (one being my husband), and two have borderline high blood pressure and are being closely monitored.

Besides medication, high blood pressure treatment usually includes weight reduction. If you're obese, you should avoid excess sodium and salt in your diet, control heavy drinking, and exercise. You should be doing most of these anyway for diabetes and for your general health.

F.Y.I. Who's at risk for hypertension?

- The incidence of severe high blood pressure is three times higher for blacks than for whites.
- The older you get, the higher your risk. (By age 74, half the U.S. population has hypertension.)
  If you're considered "obese," your risk is increased.
- If you're over 35, use oral contraceptives, and smoke, your risk is increased.
- If you have diabetes or kidney disease, your risk is high.

There are some minerals, relatively new on the hypertension scene, that may help in the treatment and possibly the prevention of hypertension:

- **Magnesium:** Eat magnesium-packed foods, such as fruits and vegetables, whole grains, and low-fat dairy items to ensure a good intake of magnesium.

- **Potassium:** A diet rich in potassium (for those without kidney damage or failure) may provide protection of the arteries for people with high blood pressure. It may also lower blood pressure a little and protect the kidneys from related damage. Potassium is the mineral that made the banana famous. But potatoes, apricots, orange and grapefruit juice, and just about any kind of fruit and vegetable not cooked in water (because some of the potassium will pass from the vegetable into the water) will add potassium to our diets. (People with a history of kidney failure should check with their doctors before increasing the intake of potassium-rich foods.)

- **Calcium:** Just when you thought it was best to avoid dairy products, evidence turns up linking decreases in systolic blood pressure (the top number in the blood pressure reading) with higher intake of calcium or calcium supplements. It seems to work the best in people with previously low intakes of calcium (below the recommended daily allowance) who also have high systolic blood pressure readings.

4. Salt movers and shakers

Here's the deal. About one in five Americans are thought to have a sensitivity to sodium (which is found in many things including salt, MSG, soy sauce, brine, broth, and any compound with the word "sodium" in it such as sodium phosphate). People who eat out and eat processed foods tend to take in a lot more sodium (and salt). The trick here is that everyone has a different level of salt that they are used to tasting in food. If you are used to quite a bit of salt/sodium in your food, lower sodium items will taste bland to you (temporarily). So restaurants and food manufacturers tend to ere in favor of the people used to tasting more salt/sodium in their food. This learned preference for salt takes about two months to unlearn. As you eat less and less salt/sodium, your taste buds become more aware of the salt and sodium that's there—but it takes time, so try and be patient.

There's not much you can do about the salt/sodium in restaurant foods and certain processed foods like turkey dogs, bacon, lunchmeats, and the occasional frozen entrée. But you can at least stop using the salt shaker.

When it comes to salt there are two types of people— the "movers" and the "shakers." The "movers" move the salt shaker to the cabinet and bring it out only if absolutely necessary. Most "shakers" (people who like to shake that salt) usually do so before even tasting the food. If this describes you, you my friend are in a bad habit. If you've got to shake something, opt for freshly ground pepper or several of the Mrs. Dash salt free seasonings. Keep in mind that one-half teaspoon of salt is worth 1,000 milligrams of sodium.

5. Type II and thin

There is a small percentage of people who have Type II diabetes but are not overweight. This describes about one in every 10 persons with Type II diabetes. Many of these people successfully manage their diabetes with oral medications (not insulin). This makes them similar to other people with Type II diabetes, but they don't have many of the other medical problems (extra weight, blood pressure, and elevate blood fats) that are common in the majority of people with Type II diabetes.

Thin people with Type II diabetes tend to be more sensitive to medications. They may need to pay attention to preventing blood sugars that are too low. It is essential that these people work with a certified diabetes educator or dietitian to fine tune their daily food plan because their greatest challenge may be to find ways to get *more* calories into their day without throwing their blood sugars off too much.

6. A diabetic on dialysis

Some people with Type II diabetes are on dialysis because their kidneys can't do their job anymore. Many of these people experience drastic swings in their blood sugars so they might need to check their blood sugars more often, particularly when they are first getting used to dialysis. You can work with a certified diabetes educator or dietitian when you first begin dialysis to help fine tune your meal plan based on your dialysis schedule. Your food plan may need to be different on days that you have and don't have dialysis.

If you are on dialysis you need to make sure you are getting enough protein to maintain your lean body mass (which keeps your metabolic rate higher) but not too much that your levels of BUN (blood urea nitrogen) are too high in between dialysis visits. Generally, you are encouraged to eat from .6 to 1.2 grams of protein per kilogram body weight per day (depending on how many times you go to dialysis a week, what type of dialysis, and other factors).

7. Syndrome X

Syndrome X, also known as the metabolic (all energy changes that take place in living cells) syndrome, is basically a collection of certain physical and medical problems. If you have or are at risk of having Type II diabetes and you are also overweight, have high blood pressure, and your serum triglyceride levels are too high, you are one of a growing group of people who have what some scientists refer to as syndrome X.

I know that, at first, it seems that high blood pressure, high triglycerides, obesity and diabetes are all separate medical problems. But it is quite possible that all of these are actually related to the same metabolic-based problem where there is a disturbance in metabolizing carbohydrates (Type II diabetes) and lipids (high serum triglycerides and low levels of the "good" or HDL cholesterol). What causes this metabolic disturbance? We don't really know, but syndrome X is generally associated with obesity. But which comes first the chicken or the egg—the obesity or the metabolic disturbances?

No matter what the cause, if this describes you, you need to know what type of eating plan tends to work best— higher carbs and lower fat or a more moderate carbohydrate and higher fat eating plan. And the winner is...The more moderate fat diet (rich in monounsaturated fats and omega-3 fatty acids but low in animal fats)—about 30 to 40 percent calories from fat. But will this make you fatter? When the calories going in are kept constant, diets slightly higher or lower in fat do not appear to result in significant weight gain. The trick to eating 30 to 40 percent calories from fat is not exceeding your required amount of energy (calories) and emphasizing monounsaturated fat and omega-3 fatty acids while limiting saturated and trans fats. (See Chapter 3 for more information on higher or lower levels of fat.)

 **Chapter 3**

Everything You Ever Wanted to Ask Your Dietitian...

Diet and Type II diabetes

It is normal for you to have lots of questions about food, your diet, and diabetes. If you could only have a couple of hours with a dietician....Well, the next best thing might be a chapter with answers to the most commonly asked questions. Read on.

Do you have a list of foods I cannot eat?
No—there isn't a list of foods you absolutely cannot eat. All foods, with smaller serving sizes, can be worked into a particular eating plan. If dietitians say you can't have something anymore, it will only make you feel deprived and angry. And you will only want to have that food more. You ultimately decide what to eat. And it is you that will learn to associate certain foods in certain amounts and in certain combinations with higher blood sugars in your particular body.

Q **I have a sweet tooth. Can I still eat some of my favorite desserts?**

If you are told you can't have something, it only makes you want it more. There is no reason why people with diabetes can't have sugar, as long as they keep a few things in mind. Bread and several other starches actually have almost the same effect on blood sugar in some people as refined sugar does. The 1994 recommendations from the American Diabetes Association basically says if you are managing your blood sugar well, then you may have some sugar—but you've got to play by a few rules:

- *Pay attention to portion sizes of sugary foods.* Keep servings moderate, like a half-cup of ice cream or three Oreo cookies.

- *Try to enjoy your dessert or high-sugar treat as part of a meal.* You will be less likely to overeat the treat if you have it with a meal and the dessert will be less likely to send your blood sugar soaring if it's paired with other foods.

- *Substitute the sugar-containing food for another carbohydrate containing food in your personal diabetes meal plan.* Otherwise you will not only increase the carbohydrates you're taking in, you'll also increase your calories.

- *Monitor your blood glucose routinely so you'll be aware of any negative effects from the sugary food.* After a certain dessert or snack (or a certain situation), you might notice a higher blood sugar an hour or so after it's eaten.

The lesson here: Go ahead and eat cake, but make it a modest slice and have it with your meal. One last bit of advice: Make sure these foods are truly satisfying, so you'll be happy with the moderate amounts.

Q **How can I do this without counting and measuring foods?**
I don't like counting and measuring either. It automatically makes you feel "different" (and not in a good way) and frankly it can take the fun out of eating. I would strongly suggest doing some counting of carbohydrate, fat and fiber grams every now and then just to sort of "check in" with how you are eating. When you compare it to blood sugars, this can be a great tool for you and your dietitian or diabetes educator. But if you really can't bring yourself to do it, the only answer is to monitor, monitor, monitor (your blood sugars that is). Monitor your blood sugar three to six times a day, study your normal diet and the resulting blood sugars, and soon you will know which foods/meals work best.

The foods that do cause high blood sugars may need to be eaten in smaller amounts each time, combined with other foods, or coordinated with a change in medication or exercise just when that specific food/meal is eaten.

Q **Should I become a vegetarian?**
A total vegetarian diet can be high in carbohydrates, making normal blood sugars harder to achieve for some. If you choose to eat this way for other reasons, make sure you plan meals carefully to keep carbohydrates in check. You will need to depend heavily on higher protein and fat plant foods like nuts and soybeans or tofu and plant foods rich in soluble fiber to help buffer the carbohydrate induced rise in blood glucose. What might appeal more to most people is not to necessarily eat a "vegetarian diet," but to just eat more plant foods.

Q Why is it important that I eat more plant foods?
"Plant foods" include fruits and vegetables, grains (such as bread, rice, pasta, and cereal), tubers (includes the potato family), and legumes (includes the beans and peas family). As you can tell from the list, these foods tend to be loaded with vitamins, minerals, fiber, and phytochemicals (plant chemicals that have health promoting properties,) most of which help protect against cancer in a variety of ways. Nutrients in plant foods also help protect our bodies from other diseases such as heart disease, stroke, and hypertension. Making plant foods take up a larger portion of our dinner plate can also help reduce obesity.

Q I've heard there is a type of fiber that is good for people with Type II diabetes. What is it?
Soluble fiber (fiber that is soluble or dissolves in water) seems to be a vital component of blood glucose control for many people. It is found in peas and beans, oats and oat bran, barley, and some fruits and vegetables. Soluble fiber leaves the stomach slowly, so it makes you feel satisfied longer. I notice that when I have beans with lunch (such as a bean burrito), I am not hungry again until dinnertime.(This is unusual because I am usually starving several hours after lunch.) Soluble fiber, which forms a gel within the intestinal tract, slows carbohydrate absorption and reduces the rise in blood glucose and insulin following the meal.

Q Are the popular very high protein, very low carbohydrate diets good for people with diabetes?
These diets aren't good for anyone but they can be dangerous to people with Type II diabetes. People with diabetes are already at high risk for kidney disease (diabetes increases the rate that the kidneys age) and excessive food protein and high blood pressure put even more

stress on the kidneys. These are all just fad diets in disguise—they aren't based on scientific and medical truths. Just think about it: Fruits and vegetables and whole grains are some of the most nutritious foods on earth, contributing vitamins, minerals, phytochemicals, and fiber. These foods are made up of mostly what?—carbohydrates. And while it is true that insulin is normally released into the blood stream when carbohydrates are eaten (in people without diabetes), the carbohydrates are stored as fat only if the calories being eaten is greater than the amount needed by the body. So carbohydrates don't automatically turn to fat unless you are eating too much.

Okay, so people say they have lost weight on these diets. The only thing that really counts is whether they were able to keep it off (and in this respect, people haven't been as lucky). People may lose weight on these diets but not because they are low in carbohydrates, but because they tend to be low in calories. People do lose weight quickly but it isn't fat they're losing right away; it's mostly body water. As you continue the diet you will lose some fat pounds but at the same time you are losing muscle tissue.

When you eat too few carbohydrates, your body automatically starts to sacrifice its protein tissue (from major organs and muscles) for energy. And when you gain the weight back it returns as body fat not muscle tissue. Over time, losing weight and gaining it back a few times causes you to get fatter and fatter and lose more and more muscle tissue. The liver and kidneys also have to work harder processing protein into energy.

Q **Are starchy foods such as pasta, potatoes, and bread fattening?**

All of these foods are high in carbohydrate calories. Carbohydrates are only fattening when we eat more calories than our body needs. But this is also the case with foods high in protein and fat (especially fat!). By including fruits and vegetables with these starches, we are more likely to keep our portions of these delicious starches reasonable. For example, when you fix pasta, add in some broccoli or carrots. When you make a sandwich with bread, have it with a piece of fruit, some melon, or a small bowl of fruit salad. With bread, you also have the opportunity to increase your daily fiber total by choosing bread that either contains whole grains or contains added soluble fiber.

Q **I'm confused. Is fat in food good or bad? I know it's bad with some diseases but I also know it helps me control my blood sugars.**
Let me tell you a story. Once upon a time all that the townspeople knew about food fat was that it tasted good and kept their bodies a little padded so they could better survive the winter and periods when food was scarce. People often cooked their food in lard or shortening. They uninhibitedly spread butter on their bread, corn, and potatoes. People delighted in drinking extra rich milk. Fatty meats and sausages were considered highly desirable. What bliss!

Over the past 10 years things have become a lot more complicated. Fat in food is feared; its mere presence has been known to inflict guilt on people. But the latest studies are showing us that some fats have a protective effect on our body in terms of heart disease and some cancers. They are also showing that there may not be a one "right" amount of fat for all people—some people may fare better with more or less fat than others. Researchers are probably going to battle this out in the years to come but in the meantime you're trying to get a better handle on your blood sugars, your weight, and your risk of heart disease.

I don't blame you for being confused. Most of us health professionals are trying to figure it all out too. Yes, having a moderate fat diet (30 to 35 percent calories from fat) seems to add up to better blood sugars for some people with Type II diabetes compared to a very lowfat diet (10 to 20 percent calories from fat.) The fat helps slow down digestion, in general, and "paces" the introduction of glucose (from carbohydrates eaten) into the blood stream. For a variety of reasons, fat also helps some people feel more satisfied after a meal or snack.

The tricky part is knowing how much is enough for the diabetic benefits but not too much that it increases your risk of other chronic diseases and weight gain. I would try to stick around the 30 to 35 percent calories from fat mark and see what effect it has on your personal blood sugars, weight, and blood lipid levels. This way you can still have about 15 to 20 percent calories from protein, leaving around 45 to 55 percent calories from carbohydrates (hopefully mostly from whole grains, beans, fruits and vegetables).

As part of this moderate fat eating plan, you absolutely *must* turn to the more heart protective fats to make up most of this "35 percent"—the omega-3 and 9 fatty acids and the monounsaturated fats. Which means using canola oil and olive oil in cooking, choosing products that contain liquid canola oil or olive oil (non-hydrogenated), including flaxseed, and enjoying a handful of nuts every now and then, and eating fish a couple times a week.

If you like eating out, these new rules could cramp your style. Most fast food places and restaurants do *not* use liquid canola and olive oil (except maybe an Italian or Mediterranean restaurant). But more on eating out in Chapter 8.

 Do blood lipids tend to improve after people with Type II diabetes switch to monounsaturated fats and omega-3 fatty acids?

Yes! Some people who achieve good blood sugar control on low-fat/high-carb diets unfortunately see their LDL "bad" cholesterol and triglycerides increase. But after adding omega-3 fatty acids and monounsaturated fats to about 30 percent calories from fat (or a little more), many people are able to improve their blood lipids without an increase in HgA1c. (The HgA1c is a blood test that is often given to people with diabetes. It measures what your blood sugars have averaged over a period of about 90 days.)

 The more I incorporate beans into my diet (which helps my blood sugar) the more gas I get. Is there anything I can do?

The fiber and some hard-to-digest complex carbohydrate in beans and legumes end up in the large intestine. The bacteria in the intestine then work on breaking down these substances, often giving off gas as a byproduct, making you feel bloated. There are a few things you can do to minimize the gaseous effects of beans. Keep your serving of beans to about one-half cup to start with and eat beans with a balanced meal (containing protein, fat and carbohydrate). There are also a couple of over-the-counter products that claim to alleviate bean digestive distress. You can give them a try by calling their 800 numbers and asking for a free sample. Try Beano (800-257-8650). It comes as a chewable tablet or liquid that is taken with beans. Or try BeSure (800-527-5200), which comes in a capsule that you take at mealtime.

 What about the advertisements I hear for foods and products that help you burn body fat fast, even while you sleep?

To burn more body fat your body requires more calories than it is taking in with food. This means exercise, building muscle, and eating a little less than your body requires. You know what they say—if it sounds too good to be true, it usually is. Anybody can tell you anything to help sell a product. To most quick and fast claims there is no real science backing it up.

You should also avoid buying weight-loss products using "speed" substances such as ephedra, ma huang, guarana, or high doses of caffeine. These may artificially increase your metabolic rate, but can be absolutely dangerous. These substances don't offer any long-term weight loss advantages, and that's what really matters. Try to avoid the temptation of a quick fix. Trimming off extra pounds takes time. Concentrate on eating healthy and exercising; this benefits your body in many different ways—trimming off extra weight is just one of them.

What is bad and good cholesterol?

A high level of LDL-cholesterol in the blood increases the risk of fatty deposits forming in the arteries, increasing the risk of heart attack. That's how LDL has gotten its nickname as the "bad" cholesterol. Elevated levels of HDL-cholesterol, on the other hand, seem to have a protective effect against heart disease, which is why it has been coined "good" cholesterol. What about "total" serum (blood) cholesterol levels? Many people think lowering *food* cholesterol is the most important step toward lowering *blood* cholesterol. Actually, eating less saturated fat has a stronger effect on lowering blood cholesterol levels. Some studies, though, have found that eating cholesterol-rich foods increases the risk of heart disease even if it doesn't increase blood cholesterol levels.

What do all those different "fatty acid" words mean?

Here are brief definitions of key fat-related ingredient and medical terms:

Cholesterol: A chemical compound manufactured in the body. It is used to build cell membranes and brain and nerve tissues. Cholesterol also helps the body make steroid hormones and bile acids. The liver makes all the cholesterol the body needs.

Dietary cholesterol: Cholesterol found in animal products that are part of the human diet. Egg yolks, liver, meat, some shellfish, and whole-milk diary products are all sources of dietary cholesterol.

Fatty acid: A molecule composed mostly of carbon and hydrogen atoms. Fatty acids are the building blocks of fat.

Fat: A chemical compound containing one or more fatty acids. Fat is one of the three main constituents of food (the others are protein and carbohydrate). It is also the principal form in which energy is stored in the body.

Hydrogenated and partially hydrogenated fat: A fat that has been chemically altered (made more *saturated* and therefore more solid) by the addition of "hydrogen" atoms. If a vegetable oil is completely saturated or "hydrogenated" it becomes a saturated fat. When a vegetable oil is partially hydrogenated, some trans fatty acids are formed (see trans fatty acid). Margarine and shortening are examples of partially hydrogenated and hydrogenated fats.

Monounsaturated fat: Fat made of "mono" unsaturated fatty acids (which are missing "one" pair of hydrogen atoms in the middle of the molecule—they have *one* unsaturated chemical bond). Monounsaturated fats are found mostly in plant and seafoods. Olive oil and canola oils are the two high monounsaturated fat oils. Monounsaturated fats tend to lower levels of LDL-cholesterol ("bad" cholesterol) in the blood.

Polyunsaturated fat: "Poly" unsaturated fats are missing more than one pair of hydrogen atoms—they have more than one unsaturated chemical bonds. Polyunsaturated fats tend to lower levels of both good cholesterol

(HDL) and bad (LDL) cholesterol in the blood. Safflower, corn, and soy oil are mostly polyunsaturated fats.

Saturated fat: A fatty acid that has the maximum possible number of hydrogen atoms attached to every carbon atom. It is "saturated" or "full" with hydrogen atoms. Saturated fats tend to raise levels of LDL-cholesterol in the blood and elevated levels of LDL-cholesterol are associated with heart disease. Saturated fats are naturally found in animal products such as butter, lard, meat, and whole milk products.

Trans fatty acids: A polyunsaturated fatty acid in which some of the missing hydrogen atoms have been put back in a chemical process called hydrogenation. Trans fatty acids are byproducts of partial hydrogenation. Trans fats may be as dangerous to our health as saturated fats, raising LDL "bad" cholesterol and total cholesterol levels.

Lipoprotein: A chemical compound made of fat and protein. Lipoproteins that have more fat than protein are called low-density lipoproteins (LDLs). Lipoproteins that have more protein than fat are called high-density lipoproteins (HDLs). Lipoproteins are found mainly in the blood where their main function is to carry cholesterol around.

Foods and blood sugars

 How and why do certain foods raise blood sugars more than others do? Pizza, for example, causes higher blood sugars than candy.
The foods we eat contain different amounts and combinations of carbohydrates, protein, and/or fat. Vegetable oils contain all fat and granulated sugar contains all carbohydrate. Other foods contain two or three of these. All of the grams of the digestible carbohydrate we eat convert to glucose while about half of the protein and 10 percent of the fat grams we eat convert to glucose after digestion.

Carbohydrate, protein, and fat show their peak effect on blood glucose at different times after a meal, too:

- Simple sugars—show their peak effect 15 to 30 minutes after the meal.
- Complex carbohydrates—One to one and a half hours after the meal.
- Protein—Three to four hours after the meal.
- Fat—Three hours after the meal.

How a particular food affects your blood glucose has to do in part with the combination of carbohydrate, protein, and fat in the food and the portion size you eat. How quickly the food is absorbed (and how quickly it affects blood glucose levels) also has to do with things like the physical form of the food, whether the food is cooked, and what blood glucose levels were at the time we ate. One trick all diabetics have up their sleeves is dietary fiber. Dietary fiber, which is not digested by the body, causes other carbohydrates in the meal to be digested and absorbed more slowly.

However, people respond differently to carbohydrates. The same meal eaten by two different people might have varying effects on blood glucose levels. And, in some people, insulin becomes less effective after they eat high animal fat meals. This can also bring on high blood sugars. The only way to know for sure how your blood sugar responds to a particular meal is to test your blood sugar before and two hours after the meal.

 What are the meals/foods that surprisingly encourage higher blood sugars than expected in some people?

Some health professionals call this "the pizza effect." So you can guess what is at the top of this list—pizza. Other foods that cause many people problems are:

- Chinese food in general (chow mein in particular).

- Ramen noodles.

- Bagels eaten plain (even one bagel can cause a problem for some). Start with half a bagel and eat it with some peanut butter or light cream cheese.

- Fried foods (such as fried chicken and French fries).

- Granola cereal (start with one-quarter cup).

- Pasta (try a one-cup serving of cooked 100 percent durum wheat semolina pasta and start the meal with a soup or salad).

- High animal protein/fat meals (including those with lots of cheese).

 Are there any foods that help prevent higher blood sugars after a meal that would normally tend to raise blood sugars?

Adding plant foods that contribute some fat and/or protein to the meal (nuts, soyfoods, olive and canola oil, flaxseed, avocado) seems to help minimize high blood sugars from notorious high carb meals. But if you have a meal high in animal fat that usually brings on high blood sugars (pizza, high fat breakfasts, etc.) loading up on fiber (soluble fiber in particular) about 10 minutes before you start the meal, may help. Higher soluble fiber plant foods will also help minimize high blood sugars from high carb meals too. As an appetizer (a little before you eat the entrée) try:

- A green salad with beans and raw vegetables.

- A cup of vegetable or bean soup.

- A small serving of oat bran or oatmeal (before a problematic breakfast).

- Other high soluble fiber vegetables or grain foods (see Chapter 4 for a list).
- Psyllium seed foods and supplements (powders without intestinal stimulants are available; pysllium is also added to a couple of breakfast cereals).

 How come I seem to have higher blood sugars after high fat meals instead of high carbohydrate meals?

Some people seem to have high blood sugars after meals particularly high in animal fats like pizza topped with sausage and pepperoni or bacon and egg breakfasts. Some researchers think that in some people (particularly certain ethnicities) insulin becomes less effective after meals laden in animal fat. If you notice this happens with you, try having smaller portions of the fatty foods and add in some plant foods (fruits, vegetables, and grains, especially those rich in soluble fiber) and see if it makes a difference. Instead of sausage and eggs and hashbrowns, try one sausage link, one egg, and pancakes or a bowl of oatmeal. Trade your four slices of "animal lover's pizza" in for:

- A few slices of "vegetable lover's" pizza. Plus...
- A green salad with kidney beans and a nice olive oil vinaigrette or a nice cup of vegetable or bean soup to go with it.

 What is the percentage of carbohydrate, fat, and protein that seems to help most people with Type II diabetes control blood sugars?

According to Certified Diabetes Educators who I spoke with, about one-third of people with Type II diabetes tend to do better with an eating plan that includes about 35 to

40 percent calories from fat (using mostly monounsaturated fats) while two-thirds tend to fair best with 25 to 30 percent calories from fat. But there are many other food factors other than the percentage of fat or carbohydrate that can influence blood sugar control such as total fiber/soluble fiber, and whether proteins and fats come mostly from vegetable sources.

Q **Who tends to do better with higher carbohydrate, lower fat meals?**

People whose insulin seems to be less effective after high saturated/animal fat meals (which seems to include Asians, Pacific Islanders, and African-Americans), tend to do better on a higher carbohydrate eating plan (especially if they are not exercising regularly). Including foods rich in soluble fiber helps many people tolerate a higher carbohydrate meal. (See Chapter 4 for more on soluble fiber.)

Q **What is a good breakfast if your blood sugars tend to be high in the morning?**

Many people with Type II diabetes have trouble with morning blood sugars, not necessarily because of what they ate for breakfast but because their "wake-up" blood sugars started high. Many people tend to be more resistant to insulin in the morning. Start by fixing yourself a nice balanced breakfast with carbohydrate, protein and fat. You can do this by adding nuts to cereal and muffins. Some people don't mind adding soy milk or almond milk to their cereals in the morning. If you are having pancakes, serve up a couple slices of turkey bacon. If you are having a bagel, add a slice of ham and cheese, a tablespoon or two of peanut butter, or one-eighth cup of light cream cheese.

Q **What about wine? Does one glass at dinner help lower blood sugars?**

A glass of red wine with dinner does seem to encourage lower blood sugars for some people, but it is very individual. For others, the opposite can happen—blood sugars seem to rise later that night. Sweeter wines tend to bring on higher blood sugars. So people tend to do better with red wines and drier wines. If you do have a glass of wine with dinner, check your blood sugar before bed and if you can try testing your blood sugar at 2 or 3 a.m. every now and then.

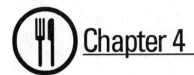

Chapter 4

The 10 Food Steps to Freedom

T rue, you need to work out an individualized eating plan with your dietitian or certified diabetes educator because what works best to normalize your blood sugars may be different from someone else. But there are 10 things all people with Type II diabetes can do to improve their health, reduce their risk of heart disease and other health risks, and make normal blood sugars more likely. That's what you will find here in the 10 Food Steps to Freedom.

I better come clean right from the get-go, though— two of the 10 "food" steps to freedom don't really involve food. One involves monitoring your blood sugar levels, and the other is to regularly exercise. They both help bring you food freedom. Monitoring blood sugars is the best way to understand how certain meals and snacks-affect your personal blood sugars—a pivotal tool in helping fine-tune your eating plan. And exercise acts like insulin in the body and can quite possibly make normal blood sugars

easier to achieve, which will give you a little more freedom in the food department. Following these 10 steps will
bring you one giant step closer to feeling better, having
normal blood sugars, and living a longer, healthier life.

Step #1: Make fiber a part of almost every meal

Fiber is the part in plant foods that humans can't
digest. Because we can't digest it, it makes it all the way
through the mouth to the stomach and then through the
small and large intestines (without being absorbed) and
out the other end. But even though it isn't absorbed, it
does all sorts of great stuff for our bodies.

There are two types of fiber. There is the kind that
doesn't dissolve in water (called insoluble fiber) which
contributes "roughage" or "bulk" to our intestinal tract.
This fiber acts like scrubbers pushing food along and helping to clean the intestinal wall as it passes through. This
is the type of fiber that is thought to help treat and prevent diverticulosis (when small pouches form in the colon
wall and can become infected) and is linked to reducing
the risk of constipation and colon cancer. It is possible
that the fiber latches onto potential carcinogens (cancer-
causing agents) within the intestines and carries them
out of the body.

The other type of fiber is particularly important if
you have Type II diabetes—soluble fiber. Soluble fiber is
different from the other type of fiber because it dissolves
in water and becomes almost gel-like. Soluble fiber does
appear to lower total serum cholesterol and LDL cholesterol levels (the higher your cholesterol levels, the more
it will help lower it). It also helps regulate blood sugars.
Because soluble fiber helps regulate blood sugars, high
fiber diets have been reported to:

- Lower postpriandial (after meals) blood sugar. (It may even improve glucose control in the meals immediately following.)
- Decrease glucose in the urine (because it helps lower blood sugars).
  Decrease insulin needs and increase tissue sensitivity to insulin.
- Reduce levels of atherosclerosis-promoting blood lipids.

It's the soluble fiber in particular that may help lessen the potential rise in blood triglycerides and other blood fats seen in some diabetics who eat a high carbohydrate diet.

One study with Type II people showed that a high-fiber eating plan reduced insulin requirements by 75 percent. Some people were able to get off insulin completely. There is one catch—soluble fiber helps lower your glucose level *after* meals, and to a lesser extent your wake-up glucose reading (fasting glucose). But this is still super helpful because we spend most of our 24-hour day in a postmeal state, right? How much fiber are we talking about? A stiff daily dose of about 30 grams of fiber.

How much fiber do we need to get our heart disease prevention benefits? About the same amount. In one study, men who ate more than 25 grams of fiber per day reduced their risk of heart disease by 36 percent compared to men who ate less than 15 grams of fiber daily. Does this sound impossible? With the right tips and recipes, and maybe a small hill of beans, some of us can hit this mark on most days.

How does soluble fiber work its magic?

The fiber slows down the absorption of other nutrients eaten at the same meal, including carbohydrates.

This slowing down may help prevent peaks and valleys in your blood sugars. (It has also been suggested that higher fiber meals improve your body's sensitivity to insulin, so it may reduce the insulin requirements in insulin-treated Type II diabetics.)

As it passes through the intestines, soluble fiber holds onto anything it can get its hands on and carries it out of the body. One of the things we know it holds onto is bile (digestive juices that the body produces using cholesterol from the body), so our body has to keep making more bile—using more cholesterol. This reduces blood cholesterol levels. Every body responds differently, but for some people combining soluble fiber with a low-fat eating plan can mean serum cholesterol reductions of 50 points or more.

There is also some evidence that soluble fiber can slow the liver's manufacture of cholesterol as well as change LDL particles so they are larger and less dense and dangerous to our arteries. Soluble fiber may also hold onto some fats and carbohydrate from the food we just ate along with the soluble fiber— "eliminating" it before it is absorbed.

Getting fiber at almost every meal

The typical American diet is anything but high in fiber. "White" grain is the American mode of operation — we eat a muffin or bagel made with white flour in the morning, have our hamburger on a white bun, then have white rice with our dinner. The more refined or "whiter" the grain-based food, the lower the fiber.

To get some fiber into almost every meal takes effort. Start by:

- Eating plenty of fruits and vegetables. Just eating five servings a day of fruits and vegetables (something we should do anyway) will get you

> to about 5 grams of soluble fiber. See Step #6 for more on fruits and vegetables.
>
> • Include some beans and bean products often (one-half cup of cooked beans will add about 2 grams of soluble fiber to your day).
>
> • Switch to less refined grains (whole grain breads and cereals, oats, brown and wild rice, barley, etc.) whenever possible.

Personally I have come to enjoy my daily fruits and vegetables. I crave beans and tofu frequently, and I don't even mind whole grain breads or using part whole wheat flour in my muffins. But I don't think I will ever get used to whole wheat pasta. That's where I personally draw the line. I do, however, buy only 100-percent semolina flour pasta (which seems to have a lower blood glucose effect compared to other pastas for many people). The point is each of us is going to draw the line in different places. Some of you might find white rice nonnegotiable while others insist on sourdough, French, or white bread. And that's okay. Just switch where you can. But if you *are* going to eat good old "white" bread, at least buy brands that have added soluble fiber sources (malted barley flour, soy fiber, and oat fiber) and other nutrients (calcium and folic acid).

Where can you find soluble fiber?

Most plant foods contain some insoluble fiber and some soluble fiber. About one-quarter to one-third of the total amount of fiber in plants is the *soluble* type—but some plant foods have more than others. The foods below are some of the richest sources of soluble fiber.

Half-cup cooked beans. Kidney beans, cranberry beans, butterbeans, canned baked beans, blackbeans, navy beans, lentils, pinto beans, great northern beans, chick peas or garbanzo, split peas, and lima beans. Some of the soluble fiber dissolves in the liquid of canned beans so if you are making a soup or stew, just stir the liquid in.

Oats and oat bran. One-half cup dry oat bran contributes 3 grams of soluble fiber. One cup of cooked oatmeal contains about 2 grams of soluble fiber. One packet of instant oatmeal contributes 1 gram of soluble fiber.

Barley. This grain has been enjoyed by other parts of the world for hundreds of years. In America you sometimes find it in soups. Even pearl barley, which has been milled, still contributes 1.8 grams of soluble fiber per three-quarters cup cooked serving.

Some fruits. Apples, mango, plums, kiwi, pears, blackberries, strawberries, raspberries, peaches; citrus fruits, including oranges and grapefruits (you'll get the most soluble fiber if you include the "pulp" and membranes dividing the fruit into sections); dried fruits including dried apricots, prunes, and dried figs.

Some vegetables. Artichokes, celery root, sweet potato, parsnip, turnip, acorn squash, potato with skin, brussels sprouts, cabbage, green peas, broccoli, carrots, French-style green beans, cauliflower, asparagus, beets.

Psyllium Seed Products. One rounded teaspoon of most psyllium products will give you about 3 grams of soluble fiber.

Give it time and lots of water

Most people's bodies seem to adjust to more fiber in their diet within about six weeks. While your body is "adjusting" you may notice a little uninvited gas. To minimize the side effects (diarrhea, abdominal pain, and flatulence) increase your fiber *slowly* and drink plenty of water (which you should be doing anyway). Soluble fiber especially absorbs water like a sponge, so drink up (only decaffienated, non-alcoholic beverages count toward the recommended eight glasses of water a day).

You can also try "Beano" pills or drops (you find it in your local drugstore) that contain an enzyme that, when taken along with beans, cabbage, broccoli, and other vegetables, helps reduce the side effects. If you are using dry beans, don't cook the beans in the soaking liquid because the gas-producing sugars leach into the water. For a handful of great bean recipes, see Chapter 6. For lists of higher fiber cereals and convenience products, see Chapter 7.

High fiber bonus for calorie watchers

Both fiber types help us feel fuller faster when they are part of the meal—discouraging overeating. When people eat meals higher in fiber, they tend to eat less. One study found people ate smaller lunches after eating high fiber breakfasts. Why? Fiber lowers insulin and insulin helps stimulate your appetite. And fiber seems to help make you feel full.

There is also some evidence that fiber can help cut calories by blocking the digestion of some of the fat, protein, or carbohydrate eaten at the same time. Either way, it's a good thing if you are overweight.

Quick ways to 30 grams of fiber

1. Get at least five servings of fruits and vegetables every day.

- Add fruit in the morning, fruit as a snack (dried fruits like dried apricots, prunes and figs are particularly high in soluble fiber), and fruit as or with dessert.

- If you drink orange or grapefruit juice, opt for the kind "with pulp" to boost your soluble fiber.

- Include a vegetable with lunch, have raw vegetables as an afternoon snack or pre-dinner appetizer, then enjoy vegetables with dinner.

2. Include a serving of beans several times a week.

- Research is showing that a diet high in legumes (beans and peas) improves all aspects of diabetes control (lowered blood sugars and improved blood lipid levels).

3. Include a high fiber cereal almost every day at breakfast or as a snack.

- Have oatmeal (or another high oat-bran food) often for breakfast, or as an evening snack.

- Switch to "whole" grains when possible such as brown or wild rice, whole wheat or whole grain bread. Use part whole wheat flour when making breads or muffins at home.

4. Perhaps include a serving of a high-fiber supplement.

- Ground flaxseed (see Step #8 for more about flaxseed).

- Bran Buds combines some less concentrated psyllium with wheat.

- About a tablespoon of 100 percent psyllium supplement with no chemical stimulants) taken with a meal once a day. Make sure you are drinking your obligatory eight glasses of water a day and *consult your doctor, dietitian or diabetes educator first*! A small number of people have an allergic reaction to it and it can also alter the absorption of other medications you may be taking. Psyllium in powdered form is recommended by one researcher who used

Sugar-Free Orange Metamucil in a study. Mix the tablespoon of the powder with juice, cereals, soups, etc. But eat or drink the mixture soon. If you don't, you'll need a spoon not a straw (soluble fiber forms a gel remember?).

Keep in mind, researchers don't know as much as they would like about the safety and value of fiber supplements taken for a long period of time and that the supplements do not include the other health promoting nutrients that foods high in fiber contribute.

Step #2: Count carbohydrates

Every now and then, count your carbohydrates to make sure you are hitting your desired amounts per meal/snack (and to compare to your blood sugars).

It isn't that carbohydrates are bad. It's just that you need to know what amount of carbohydrates your body can tolerate (at different times of the day) given your body, medication, and exercise schedule.

Having to count anything everyday gets tiresome real fast. Having to write down what you eat makes you feel

---

F.Y.I. **Beans for lunch**

Eating beans produces a slow rise in blood sugars. The "gel" formed in the intestines makes the passage of glucose from food into the cells go in slow motion. Lunch is a very strategic time to eat beans because it will help pace your glucose absorption from food. It will keep insulin levels low, which may prevent overeating. Later in the day, I did notice when I was pregnant that the only lunch that would keep me from becoming absolutely ravenous mid-afternoon was a bean burrito.

as though you are being punished. But the truth is, writing all this stuff down is one of the best ways to manage your diabetes. Keeping track of the food you eat and how your body reacted to it will help you understand what you can do better next time. It can pinpoint your particular trouble spots and your best strategies to combat them.

For example, if you find your blood sugar tends to get too high after you eat pizza, you can try eliminating the fatty meat toppings, eating one slice less, and having some green salad with vegetables and kidney beans instead. Will this lower you blood sugar response to pizza? Take your blood sugar one and a half hours later and find out.

The act of keeping a food/blood sugar diary helps many people reduce their total calories. This is an added bonus to people with diabetes who are also trying to trim off a few extra pounds. I know it's hard, but try to think positively about keeping your diary. Once you figure out what works best for your body, and your blood sugars become consistently normal, you won't have to keep your food diary every single day. It's a good idea to check in every once in a while though, especially if your blood sugars begin to change.

Most of the commercial food diaries available leave a space only to tabulate grams of carbohydrate. I designed the following *A Day At A Glance* to help you tabulate grams of carbohydrate plus grams of fat and fiber. Knowing the grams of fat and fiber helps complete the picture. You might find that it's the really high fat meals that cause you trouble or you might find that a certain amount of fat grams seems to help normalize your blood sugars. You might discover that your blood sugars are better when your meal/snack contains a high fiber food.

A Day At A Glance includes a space to record how hungry you were when you ate. There is a space to record your blood sugar, your medication, the minutes you exercised and

A Day at a Glance

Blood Sugar Measurements

_____

_____

6 a.m. 8 a.m. 10 a.m. 12 p.m. 2 p.m. 4 p.m. 6 p.m. 8 p.m. 10 p.m. 12 a.m. 2 a.m.

Insulin or Oral Measurements
(record units or number of tablets taken at what times)

_____

_____

6 a.m. 8 a.m. 10 a.m. 12 p.m. 2 p.m. 4 p.m. 6 p.m. 8 p.m. 10 p.m. 12 a.m. 2 a.m.

Activity (minutes)

_____

_____

6 a.m. 8 a.m. 10 a.m. 12 p.m. 2 p.m. 4 p.m. 6 p.m. 8 p.m. 10 p.m. 12 a.m. 2 a.m.

Meals/Snacks   Day:_____ Date: ___/___/___

meal/snack	carbs fat fiber	hunger level

meal/snack	carbs fat fiber	hunger level

meal/snack	carbs fat fiber	hunger level

meal/snack	carbs fat fiber	hunger level

(*Hunger level: 4=very hungry, 3=moderately hungry, 2=somewhat hungry, 1=not really hungry) when. All this information will help your dietitian or diabetes educator fine-tune your eating plan.

Step #3: Emphasize heart protective fats

Emphasize heart protective fats (monounsaturated fats and omega-3 fatty acids) and count fat grams for the right balance for your meals/snacks.

You might think food fat is food fat. But as I explained earlier, there are actually three types of fats in food—saturated fatty acids, polyunsaturated fatty acids, and monounsaturated fatty acids and one of them is better for you than the others. The monounsaturated fats do not seem to promote heart disease, plaquing in the arteries, and cancer like the saturated fats and polyunsaturated fats appear to. It's a no-brainer then to start using and eating more monounsaturated fats and definitely less saturated fat.

There are basically two common oils which both contain mostly monounsaturated fats—canola oil and olive oil. They each offer additional and different health benefits (you'll find out what those are below) so I personally use both.

There are certain recipes or foods that I eat that require butter, but only if it is truly the best type of fat for that particular food. Even then, I will use the least amount I can. When I can you bet I switch to canola or olive oil or canola margarine. In most sautéing circumstances, I can use canola or olive oil. In many baking recipes such as some cakes, muffins, even pie crust, I can switch to canola oil. If the cookie or cake recipe calls for creaming the shortening or butter with sugar, then usually I can use my favorite canola margarine (Canoleo 100-percent Canola margarine distributed by Spring Tree Corp. in Brattleboro, Vermont). See Chapter 7 for more information.

Canola oil

You may have heard that canola is a "good" fat—that it contains mostly monounsaturated fat. You may have even heard that it is one of the few plant sources of omega-3 fatty acids. But how much would you need to

---

F.Y.I. Omega-3 fatty acids

Researchers are still trying to find out as much as they can about omega-3 fatty acids. So far it looks like a win-win-win situation. Omega-3 fatty acids have been linked to lowering both blood pressure and serum trig-lyceride levels, preventing blood clots and possibly increasing HDL-good cholesterol levels. They have also been shown to slow or prevent cancerous tumor growth as well as reducing symptoms of inflammatory diseases such as rhuematoid arthritis. The two particular cancers that omega-3s may help prevent are colon and possibly breast cancer.

Omega-3 fatty acids can be found in all sorts of fish, the fattier the better. My personal favorite fish sources are salmon, canned albacore tuna packed in spring water, striped bass, and pacific halibut, but you can also find them in anchovies, sardines, herring, blue-fish, mackerel, mullet, and shark.

Some plant foods contain alpha-linolenic acid which the body can partially convert to an omega-3 fatty acid. You will find alpha-linolenic acid in wal-nuts, walnut oil, flaxseed, rapeseed (used to make canola oil), soybeans, spinach, and mustard greens.

---

consume to get a potentially beneficial dose of omega-3 fatty acids? I asked researchers at Best Foods, who make Mazola's Canola Oil, to send me the actual fatty acid breakdown for one tablespoon of canola oil. I was delighted to find that just one tablespoon contained about 1.5 grams omega-3 fatty acids (about the same amount found in three-and-a-half ounces of cooked salmon). A tablespoon also contains 9 grams of omega-9 fatty acids (oleic acid, a monounsaturated fat which may reduce the development of breast carcinomas) and 7 milligrams of mixed tocopherols (a group of antioxidants which includes vitamin E, alpha-tocopherol).

Canola oil has a neutral flavor and can be heated to high temperatures so I like to use canola oil in baking and frying recipes.

Olive oil

The people in the Mediterranean region have been studied lately because they have surprisingly low rates of heart disease and yet their typical diet is not terribly low in fat. Their cuisine includes abundant seafood, use of olives and olive oil, and fruits, vegetables, and nuts. We now know that all of those foods have health benefits for our body—including olive oil.

Olive oil does not contain omega-3 fatty acids like canola oil, but the majority of fatty acids in olive oil are still the more beneficial monounsaturated fats. Olive oil contains fatty acids; 56 to 83 percent of these acids are specifically oleic acid (an up and coming omega-9 fatty acid). Canola oil also contributes more vitamin E than olive oil. But there is something that olive oil adds to your diet that canola oil doesn't—potentially protective phytochemicals found in olives.

Olive oil has a marvelous distinctive range of possible flavors, ranging from peppery to pungent, so I like to use olive oil in my Italian recipes, cold salad type of recipes, marinades and vinaigrettes.

Why count fat grams?

It is helpful to count fat grams because the issue of food fat for most people with Type II diabetes can be a little tricky. You want enough fat to help balance carbohydrates, but not too much. The only way to know what level of fat grams works best for you at what time of day, is to count them every now and then. Take a look at your food diary and see what level of fat tends to produce better blood sugars at certain times of day.

Everybody is different but most people with Type II diabetes handle carbohydrates better when they are eaten alongside some protein and fat. Fat helps lower the blood glucose response of the other foods it is eaten with. So, "some" fat is definitely a good thing—especially if it is rich in the more protective type of fats (monounsaturated fat, omega-3 and omega-9 fatty acids). What we are really talking about is a balancing act—pairing your carbohydrate-rich foods (breads, grains, starches, fruits, sweets, etc.) with foods that contribute some protein and fat.

It's a good idea, when you are trying to figure out which foods and food combinations you do best with, to count fat grams along with carbohydrate grams. For many people with Type II diabetes, some fat helps, but meals that are too high in fat (especially highly saturated animal fats) can have terrible consequences on after-meal blood sugars. In some people, meals high in animal fats make the body very resistant to insulin. Breakfasts like sausage and eggs or your typical pepperoni and sausage pizza can be blood glucose nightmares to many.

What this means in food terms is that you need to:

- Switch to using olive oil and canola oil (instead of other vegetable oils) when possible.

- Eat more fish.

- Eat less animal fat by choosing leaner meats and lower fat dairy products and by eating plant protein (from soy, beans, and vegetables) instead of animal protein sometimes.

- Limit foods that contain high amounts of hydrogenated and partially hydrogenated oils (the hydrogenation process produces trans fatty acids which are as damaging (if not more damaging) to our hearts and arteries than saturated fat.

- Figure out what to do about butter or margarine. There are some better tasting tub margarines that list liquid canola oil or olive oil as the first ingredient. If you use butter, fine. Just use less and use canola oil or olive oil in cooking instead when you can.

Cooking with the right fats

If a recipe calls for vegetable oil, just use canola oil. If it calls for vegetable oil and you think the flavor in olive oil would compliment the dish, and the oil wouldn't be heated to a high temperature (olive oil starts smoking and breaking down at higher temperatures), then you can even use olive oil instead. But what about the recipes that call for shortening, stick butter or margarine? That gets a little trickier.

If you are using a lower fat recipe from the start, that helps because whatever fat you are using is at least being added in smaller amounts. (Check out a few of my cookbooks for some great reduced fat recipes, or my national column called "The Recipe Doctor." Also, check out my Web site, recipedoctor.com.)

Sometimes I still use butter because it may truly be the best fat for that recipe; I just cut it down as far as I can (substituting in other high-flavor/high-moisture ingredients. If butter isn't that essential to the recipe and the original recipe calls for beating the butter, margarine or shortening in a mixer, usually with sugar then eggs, you can switch to a margarine with liquid canola oil as the first ingredient. Sometimes you can get away with beating part canola oil and part fat-free cream cheese or sour cream in place of the original fat. If you are sautéing something in a pan, you can easily switch to canola or olive oil and you can probably use less than in the original recipe, especially if you are using nonstick pans.

Start collecting recipes that your family like that call for olive or canola oil. I made up a reduced-fat pie crust recipe that uses canola oil. I now use salad dressings that contain canola or olive oil for my vinaigrette-dependent recipes (such as green salad and pasta salad). These are the kinds of changes you can start making right now.

Step #4: Keep saturated fat and cholesterol low

If monounsaturated fat is now "in" then saturated fat is definitely "out." You'd be hard pressed to find someone who doesn't know that Americans need to eat less saturated fat. High amounts of saturated fat are clearly associated with heart disease. More specifically, saturated fat has been shown to raise bad cholesterol (LDL) and triglycerides in the blood. Obviously eating less saturated fat is good, solid advice. Giving that advice is easy, following it is the tough part—especially here in America.

Saturated fat is synonymous with typical American food. It's in hamburgers and French fries, pizza, hot dogs and even apple pie.

It doesn't matter whether you find your blood sugars improve with a low or moderate fat eating plan. Either way, saturated fat and food cholesterol need to be low. Cholesterol should be limited to 300 milligrams or less a day and saturated fat is supposed to contribute no more than 10 percent of the total calories.

Saturated fat sources

The biggest contributor of saturated fat and cholesterol in the American diet is the meat group, which includes beef, processed meats, eggs, poultry and other meats. In general, if you choose leaner meats (lower in fat), use egg substitute in place of half the eggs (a good rule of thumb), and take the skin off poultry, you will lower the amount of saturated fat and cholesterol.

The runner up to meat is the milk group (includes cream and cheese), which is the second largest saturated fat contributor. Select lower fat dairy options and you are guaranteed less saturated fat and cholesterol.

Saturated fat is found in other animal fats too such as butter, ice-cream, lard, bacon, anything made with coconut and palm oil, and vegetables oils that have been "hydrogenated" as is the case with stick margarine and shortening. Many of the packaged foods we buy like crackers, cookies, snack foods, frozen fried foods, pastries, etc., contain hydrogenated oils.

Where to cut cholesterol

Plant foods do not contain cholesterol. So we find cholesterol only in animal foods. Where you find high amounts of fat in animal products, generally cholesterol isn't far behind. Food sources highest in cholesterol are egg yolks, organ meats (especially liver), whole-fat dairy products and higher fat meats. There are a few fish sources that are a bit higher in cholesterol like shrimp and squid, but they are low in fat and saturated fat so I wouldn't worry too much about the occasional shrimp cocktail or calamari you enjoy in restaurants.

Avoiding organ meats is the easy part. Buying skinless chicken is simple too. And I have personally found it no problem at all to switch to lowfat milk and yogurt and reduced fat cheese and sour cream. I generally use half real eggs and half egg substitute when I'm cooking. Muffins, cakes, quiches, even omelets still turn out terrific.

Big or little results

Keep in mind some people show big changes in their serum cholesterol after dietary cholesterol and saturated fat have been increased or decreased, while others show little changes. Blame or thank your genetics. Some people are more sensitive to the cholesterol-raising effects of foods high in saturated fat and cholesterol than others.

Step #5: Calories do count

Why do some people need to eat so much of the fat-free and light products? Could it be, perhaps, that these foods are less satisfying, so we eat more in hopes of becoming more satisfied? Just a thought. Perhaps we also tend to eat more because we think they can do no harm no matter what the quantity. Don't get me wrong, I'm a fan of quite a few of the better-tasting reduced fat products. But remember, the benefits of eating lower fat and calorie products are quickly lost with larger serving sizes.

Mind over matter

How does thinking we are eating something very low fat or fat free affect our overall intake? In one study, women ate more at lunch when they ate a yogurt labeled low fat than they did after eating the yogurt labeled high fat—even though the yogurts contained the same number of calories. Perhaps this has something to do with women paying less attention to their actual hunger and more attention to controlling their intake.

You still need to listen to your hunger cues. If you are hungry, you should eat. When you are no longer hungry, but comfortable, you should stop eating. In terms of counting though, it is helpful if you are counting what you eat so that you can look back on your after-meal blood sugars and get an idea of how your body handled that particular amount and combination of foods for next time.

Step #6: Eat more fruits and vegetables

Starting your meals and/or snacks with fruits and vegetables is a trick I've learned with my family. If you start your meal by enjoying fruits and vegetables, you'll be sure to get some and they will help fill you up so you won't be as likely to overeat the meat or entrée. Eating at a pizza parlor is a perfect example. While you are waiting for your pizza, relax and enjoy a nice green salad with tomato, kidney beans, and other vegetables (making sure to keep regular dressings to about a tablespoon). You'll find that you won't eat as much pizza. If you eat the salad at the same time you eat your pizza, you are more likely not to eat as much salad and vegetables.

There are so many health reasons to eat more fruits and vegetables; they contain fiber, vitamins and minerals, antioxidants, phytochemicals, and most are naturally low in fat, sugar and sodium. The sad truth is, we already know this. We just don't get around to eating enough fruits and vegetables most days. Some people say it is because they aren't as convenient as snack foods and fast food. Others say they simply aren't in the habit. Well, whatever your reason, the time to change this is now.

Making fruits and vegetables habit-forming

I think we would all eat more fruits and vegetables if we just had a mother taking care of us. We need someone to remember to buy the fruits and vegetables, someone to take the time to turn them into beautiful fruit salads or green salads, snack trays, and garnishes or tasty side dishes to our entrees. All this takes time, talent, and love. Here are some ways to make fruits and vegetables a little more convenient.

- Pack your desk or car with your favorite dried fruits; they will keep for weeks.
- Buy baby carrots and celery sticks and put them out before dinner with a quick dip (mix some light or fat free sour cream with Hidden Valley Ranch dressing powder or onion dip powder to taste).
- Take time Sunday or at the beginning or end of the work week to make a large spinach salad or vegetable fortified lettuce salad, and just store it (without dressing) in an airtight container. You can have crisp, wonderful salad as a snack or with your lunch or dinner for the next few days.
- Every few days make a point of going to your supermarket and picking out the best tasting and freshest in-season fruits. Put them out as a snack for the family. Add a few slices or wedges of fruit to each lunch or dinner plate.

- With a few chops of a knife, you can turn a few pieces of fruit into a beautiful fruit salad. Drizzle lemon, pineapple or orange juice over the top and toss to coat the fruit with it (the vitamin C helps prevent browning).
- Buy your favorite fruits in the winter frozen or canned in juice or light syrup.
- Stock up your refrigerator at work and home with your favorite fruit juices (make sure they are all 100 percent juice). You can often buy them in individual servings so you can grab them as soon as you are running out the door.
- Make a point to include a vegetable with your lunch.
- Make sure you enjoy vegetables when you eat out at a restaurant or deli.

For a list of fruits and vegetables rich in soluble fiber refer back to Step #1.

Step #7: Avoid eating large meals

Eating more often, but smaller amounts at a time, is a good idea for every single American but can be particularly helpful for people with Type II diabetes.

What small meals do for blood sugar levels

Small meals eaten about every two and a half to three hours translate into more stable blood sugars throughout the day. Smaller meals generally result in smaller blood glucose responses, requiring less insulin and improving blood glucose control in people with Type II diabetes.

It makes sense that the bigger the meal, the larger the number of calories eaten from carbohydrate, fat, and protein, and the higher the blood levels of those nutrients will be after the "large" meal. Large meals also zap you of your after-meal energy. If you've had a large meal, a nap is usually not far behind. But if you eat smaller meals you will feel more energetic throughout your day. (Smaller, lower fat meals don't stay in the stomach long; they move quickly to the intestines.) If you feel "light" on your feet, you will be more likely to be physically active too. The more physically active, the more calories you will burn going about your day. Don't forget that exercise and activity acts like insulin in the body too.

Other benefits of small meals

If you don't want to eat this way to help your diabetes, then do it for these other great reasons:

- Your brain and body require a constant supply of energy in the blood. Eating smaller, more frequent meals is more likely to keep your blood sugar (and energy) stable—preventing low blood sugar levels (which can trigger headaches, irritability, food cravings, or overeating in susceptible people.)

F.Y.I. **How soon after a meal does your blood glucose peak**

Depending on the exact composition and size of your meal, your blood glucose (blood sugar) begins to rise 30 to 60 minutes after eating and peaks about one-and-a-half to two hours after the meal.

- Eating smaller, more frequent meals is great for appetite control. The more stable blood sugars keep us from getting overly hungry, which can lead to overeating or making high-sugar or high-fat food choices.

- One study observed that obesity was less common in people who ate more frequent meals. People who eat smaller, more frequent meals are less likely to overeat at any meal. Larger meals flood your bloodstream with fat, protein, and carbohydrate calories and your body has to get rid of any extra calories. What does this have to do with being overweight? All extra calories can be converted to body fat for energy storage.

- This is still being investigated but it is possible that this eating style may help lower serum cholesterol. It stands to reason that by avoiding large meals you also prevent quick rises of serum triglycerides that typically follow large, particularly fatty meals.

- Burn more calories digesting, absorbing, and metabolizing food just by eating more often. The body burns calories when it digests and absorbs food. Every time we eat, the digestion process kicks in. If we eat six small meals instead of two large ones, we start the digestive process three times more often every single day—burning more calories. Calories burned by activating the metabolism can amount to about 5 to 10 percent of the total calories we eat in a day.

- It's physically more comfortable to eat smaller meals. You aren't weighed down by a large meal in your stomach.

How frequent should the "smaller" meals be?

Experts have not yet determined the ideal eating pattern for people with diabetes but so far it seems that the closer together the meals are, the better the results. The longer the gap between a previous meal or snack and dinner, for example, the larger the dinner typically ends up being.

If you eat a small breakfast, have a midmorning snack, a light lunch, then an afternoon snack, and a light dinner and maybe a nighttime snack—it adds up to six small meals for the day. Until researchers know more, the best advice I can give you is to space your meals according to your individual schedule, when you tend to get hungry, and in line with your blood glucose levels.

Fight the urge to eat at night

We burn 70 percent of our calories as fuel during the day, but when do many Americans eat the majority of their calories? During the evening hours. Eating small meals can break this habit. If you eat small meals throughout the day, eat when you're hungry and stop when you're "comfortable," it should be easier to avoid eating large dinners and evening desserts and snacks. Keep in mind that what you eat in the evening will be hitting your blood stream pretty much around the time you are getting in your jammies. It isn't as though you are eating to fuel a marathon or anything.

When a bedtime snack is in order

If you eat an early dinner, you may need to eat a small bedtime snack. Choose something you tolerate well like an apple or small bowl of oatmeal. I know it's hard to believe, but this helps reduce early morning blood glucose levels.

Easier said than done

Our whole society is based on three meals a day—with dinner typically being the largest meal of the day. This is a hard habit to break. If you eat out often, it becomes particularly difficult not to eat a large meal. Restaurants tend to serve large meals and that's all there is to it. It requires extra diligence at restaurants to eat only half your meal and save the rest for later. If you are having spaghetti, you could eat the salad and half your entrée, then have the garlic bread and the rest of your spaghetti later or the next day. I'm not saying it isn't going to be difficult—but it can be done.

Step #8: Improving diet with supplements

When you walk into a vitamin supplement store you're a sitting duck. Remember, the business of selling supplements is a big and lucrative one. The more pills they can talk you into, the thicker their wallets. Now don't start

---

F.Y.I. If you are on insulin or other medications...

Your meals and medications need to fit together well. For example, meals need to be spaced according to the type of insulin you are taking and its period of peak action. It is important that you discuss your new eating schedule (eating smaller, more frequent meals) with your dietitian or certified diabetes educator first because this person can help modify your medications accordingly.

getting your checkbook out. The supplements I'm talking about shouldn't run you very much at all. In fact you can buy them at your local drugstore or supermarket.

Start with a good multivitamin plus minerals

One of the best things you can do for yourself is to take a good multivitamin with minerals—such as Centrum. (If you are female and don't have a menstrual period anymore, no matter what your age, you might be better off with Centrum Silver which contains less iron.)

Taking a multivitamin with minerals is like having nutrition insurance. We feel better knowing that if we aren't getting enough in our food, at least we are getting some from our multivitamin. Multivitamins have come a long way and many are very balanced and complete and even include recommended amounts of up-and-coming minerals like chromium, selenium, and boron. A two-month supply will cost you about $3 a month.

Many of the vitamins and minerals you will find in your top notch multivitamin with minerals may actually help your diabetes:

Chromium. This mineral might make cells more receptive to insulin. Some experts say it does decrease HbA1c levels (200 mcg several times a day) and some say it doesn't. More studies are needed because of chromium's unproven benefits and unknown risks. You can get about 65 to 120 mcg of chromium in your multivitamin.

Magnesium. A deficiency of this mineral may help contribute to hypertension. If a person's diet is deficient it may also make cells more resistant to insulin. A multivitamin usually contains about 100 mg (25 percent of the RDA).

Antioxidants. Some researchers think people with diabetes use up their antioxidant stores more quickly, increasing their requirements (sort of like smokers do).

They think this happens with diabetes because the disease creates more free radicals, which use up the vitamins. With high levels of glucose in the blood, it is thought that some of the glucose molecules bind onto proteins and lipids (called glycosylation) making them more susceptible to oxidation. This oxidation process generates more free radicals.

Vitamin C. Some researchers have found that 250 to 500 milligrams of vitamin C can reduce glycosylation. Most multivitamins contain at least 60 milligrams.

Vitamin E. This antioxidant has been associated with many heart disease prevention benefits at the level of 200 to 400 IU per day, but some researchers say that supplementation may also improve blood sugars. Most multivitamins contain 30 to 45 IU (Centrum Silver contains 45 IU).

Selenium is an important antioxidant. Some multivitamins contain about 20 mcg per pill.

Folic acid. This acts like an antioxidant in the body. It is known (along with the B vitamins) for assisting in the lowering of elevated homocysteine levels in the body (high levels of homocysteine are associated with increased risk of heart disease). Two groups of people are known to have problems with elevated homocysteine levels: people with a rare genetic problem that causes early heart attacks and people with diabetes. More needs to be known about the benefits of folic acid for people with diabetes but one researcher reported that folic acid may help with vascular disease in people with Type II diabetes. Your typical basic multivitamin contains 400 mcg.

Reading the label

When you are shopping for your multivitamin with minerals ask yourself these questions:

Does it contain the known antioxidants?

Look for vitamin A (some of which is beta carotene), vitamin E, vitamin C and selenium

Does it contain chromium?

Even though we don't yet have a daily recommended amount for the mineral chromium, it is important that your supplement have at least the minimum Recommended Daily Allowance—50 mg—because it is one of the minerals we seem to need more of as we age.

Does it contain all the B vitamins and folic acid. Does it contain more B-12 than other multivitamins? People over 50 often don't absorb enough B-12 from the foods they eat. Many of the multivitamins formulated for people over 50 contain more B-12.

Does it contain 100 percent of the daily value for most of the vitamins and minerals and if it doesn't, does it have a good reason to include more or less?

There are some exceptions. Biotin will only be at 10 percent daily value because it is very expensive, and you won't find calcium or magnesium in amounts much greater than 25 percent daily value because they add so much bulk. (If they did put 100 percent of the daily value they would look more like horse pills!)

How much iron does it contain?

If you are still menstruating, you will mostly likely need the multivitamins with 100 percent daily value of iron. If you are female and are no longer menstruating (or no longer have a uterus) choose the multivitamins that contain the lowest amount of iron. At this time, your body can't get rid of any excess iron and so it can accumulate in tissues and organs causing problems. Centrum silver contains 4 mg of iron compared to regular Centrum which contains 18 mg.

How much of the "bone building" micronutri-ents—calcium, magnesium and vitamin D—does it contain? Does it include enough vitamin D?

As we age, we lose the ability to make vitamin D through our skin. The daily recommended intake (DRI) for vitamin D is 400 IU for age 51 to 70. Most multivitamins contain 400 IU.

Supplementing vitamin E

Many researchers are recommending about 400 IU of vitamin E for potential immune and heart disease prevention benefits. The better supplements contain only 30 to 45 IU. In the best of nutritional circumstances you can hope to take in only about 30 IU from food, leaving a gap of over 300 IU. You can find mixed tocopherol and vitamin E supplements at most grocery or drug stores at about $2 per one-month supply.

Warning: The beneficial anti-clotting effect of vitamin E could pose a danger for people on blood-thinning medications (anticoagulants). If you are on any medications affecting blood clotting, you probably shouldn't take vitamin E supplements, but check with your doctor. When you are taking an aspirin a day (to help keep the cardiologist away), which also has an anticoagulant effect, you aren't usually taking enough of it to make vitamin E a problem. But if you are taking high doses of a pain reliever for chronic pain, talk to your doctor first about vitamin E supplements.

One powerful antioxidant

Alphalipoic acid is being billed by several researchers as a very strong antioxidant that helps fight insulin resistance and neuropathy. That's quite a tall order. Early studies are showing that it is indeed useful for people with diabetic neuropathy (nerve damage). One study in lean and obese people with Type II diabetes found lower fasting blood sugars in both groups when 600 milligrams were taken twice a day. There were more drastic changes, however, in the lean group. There aren't many studies on alphalipoic acid yet but so far the results seem consistent. If you are interested in this antioxidant supplement, you absolutely need to work closely with your diabetes educator because it could potentially lower blood sugars and you need to be closely monitored.

Try flaxseed

If you haven't heard of flaxseed yet, trust me you will. I predict flaxseed will be to the 21st century what wheat germ was to the 60s. It is just now being studied in humans, mostly for its blood lipid lowering benefits and tumor-reducing properties with some types of cancer. (It seems to be so effective in reducing estrogen and lowering breast cancer risk that it is now being tested clinically to shrink breast cancer tumors before surgery on women just diagnosed with breast cancer.) We will know much more about flaxseed's health benefits in 10 more years. But that is then and this is now.

What is it about the flaxseed that might be responsible for all this? We know that flaxseed is an extraordinary source of the phytoestrogen called lignans, containing 75 to 800 times as much as other plant sources. Lignans are also considered to act as antioxidants, protecting healthy cells from chance meetings with free radicals in the body.

Flaxseed is also packed with the plant form of omega-3 fatty acids, alpha-linolenic acid. In fact, about half of the oil in flaxseed is alpha-linolenic acid. It is possible the fish form of omega-3 is more powerful in the body, but it looks like the plant form offers benefits, too. The omega-3 in flaxseed help prevent blood clots that might lead to heart attacks, according to University of Toronto nutrition researcher, Stephen Cunnane, Ph.D. The omega-3s do this by helping make platelets (a component in the blood) less likely to stick together, causing a chain reaction that leads to a blood clot.

Flaxseed is at the very least a good source of soluble fiber (the type of fiber that blends with water to form a gel-like mixture in the intestines) which may help lower cholesterol and blood sugar levels. When women in Cunnane's study added about two tablespoons of ground flax to their daily diet for four weeks, their total cholesterol fell 9 percent and their LDL (bad cholesterol) dropped 18 percent (while HDL—"good cholesterol"—stayed the same). These same results were also found in a different study conducted by researchers in the United States.

Flaxseed may also make our arteries more flexible, something that would potentially lead to a decrease risk of heart attack and stroke, after supplementing your diet with it for just one month. You've heard of "hardening of the arteries"—a stiffening of blood vessel walls caused by high blood pressure, diabetes, and/or atherosclerosis? Well, flaxseed may help make the arteries less "hard." More research needs to be done on this, but so far so good.

Once you grind the seeds (and you'll want to because the body enzymes can get to the beneficial chemicals better this way) it is highly perishable (lasting only 30 days—and that's if refrigerated). If you opt for flaxseed oil you will want to take about one to two tablespoons per day and it will keep for only 30 days (refrigerated). You can't cook or bake with it (heat makes it rancid) and the oil doesn't contain the beneficial lignans and fiber because they are both removed in the process of making the oil. Since we want all the benefits from flaxseed, I recommend buying whole or ground flaxseeds, not flaxseed oil.

You will find the seeds (often in bulk bins) in health food stores. If you buy them whole, you'll need to store them in the refrigerator and grind them up yourself, in a

F.Y.I. How much flax is enough?

Some researchers say one level teaspoon is enough, others recommend one tablespoon. Certainly working up to a teaspoon of flaxseed a few times a week is a moderate approach , until more is known on the ideal daily dose.

If flaxseed had a nutrition information label it might look something like this:

1 tablespoon:

Calories: 48

Protein: 1.9 g

Carbohydrates: 3.3 g

Total fat: 3.3 g

Omega-3 fatty acids: 1.8 g

Monounsaturated fat: 0.7 g

Saturated fat: 0.3 g

Fiber: 2.7 g (1/3 of which is soluble)

Cholesterol: 0 mg

Folic acid: 27 mcg (7 percent daily value)

Magnesium: 35 mg (9 percent daily value)

Phosphorus: 48 mg

Potassium: 66 mg

Total lignans (phytoestrogens): 6,600 micrograms

Warning: Some people are highly allergic to flax, so start with one-quarter teaspoon a day and increase the amount gradually if you don't have a reaction. Another reason you want to start off slowly is that flaxseed, which is high in fiber, can cause gassiness and bloating if you aren't used to it.

spice or coffee bean grinder—perhaps a few days' supply at a time. (I recommend having a designated flax grinder for this.) Store the ground seeds in a Ziplock bag in the refrigerator and scoop out one to two teaspoons, which you can then stir into some juice, sprinkle over some hot or cold cereal, or whip up in a breakfast smoothie a few times a week. You can also bake a daily ration (or half a ration) of flaxseed into each serving of bread or muffin.

You might even be able to find a product called "Fortified Flax" which is a preground flaxseed (that looks like cornmeal). It is fortified with nutrients like vitamin C and E to stabilize it against oxidation which keeps it from going rancid. Once a package of preground flaxseed is opened, keep it refrigerated, and whatever you don't use in 6 months, throw away.

But how does it taste? You won't mind the sprinkle or two. Flaxseed has a nice nutty taste to it. In the words of flaxseed researcher Stephen Cunnane, "There's nobody who won't benefit from adding flaxseed to his or her diet." (Except those with a flaxseed allergy.)

Step #9: Monitor your blood sugars

Keeping your blood glucose as near normal as possible protects your body from diabetic complications further down the line. Measuring your blood sugar levels on a fairly regular basis, then, is a necessary step toward tightly controlling your blood sugar. Measuring your blood sugars will tell you whether you are meeting your treatment goals and whether the agreed-upon treatments (diet, exercise, or pharmacological) are working.

You are hopefully working with a dietitian or diabetes educator who is helping you personalize your eating plan. Logging in your food, blood sugars, medications and exercise per day shows your dietitian or diabetes educator how your blood sugar is being affected from day to day. This person can then work with you to fine-tune your diabetes care plan by adjusting medications, changing your desired amount of carbohydrate grams, and encouraging activity at certain times.

About an hour and a half after eating you will know whether your blood sugar is within normal limits, high, or low. This is your greatest tool. Use it. Each person reacts a little differently to each food, combinations of foods, and amount of those foods. The only way you can learn your own personal reaction to a particular meal is to test your blood sugar an hour and half after eating. Once you begin testing and recording your blood sugar levels, you can look back to your records for clues on why your readings are what they are. Look for clues in three areas:

1. Food and diet. (What foods and how much?)
2. A change in your exercise or activity schedule. (Did you exercise at your usual time for the usual length?)
3. Medication. (Did you take the proper amount of medication at the proper time?)

Make sure someone on your health care team clearly demonstrates how to measure your glucose and how to record it so it can be referred to easily at follow-up visits.

Step #10: Make exercise fun, and do it every day!

When you exercise regularly you just plain feel better. You burn more calories and you increase your muscle mass, which increases your metabolic rate. And that's just the beginning. Exercising will help decrease blood sugar levels and possibly the dose of insulin you need to take (if you take insulin). It will decrease blood cholesterol levels and bone loss while improving your circulation, heart function and your ability to deal with stress.

Make exercise a priority, please! Start making it a habit to exercise. Get a schedule going, like walking with a neighbor on Tuesdays and Thursdays and going to an exercise class on Mondays and Wednesdays.

Recommendations for exercise

If you are currently sedentary and you want to start exercising just enough to improve your risk factors for chronic diseases, exercise:

Frequency: 2 to 3 times a week
Intensity: 40% maximum heart rate
Duration: 15 to 30 minutes

If you want to be physically fit, exercise:
Frequency: 4 times a week.
Intensity: 70 to 90% maximum heart rate.
Duration: 15 to 30 minutes.

If you want specifically to lose weight, exercise:
Frequency: 5 times a week.
Intensity: 45 to 60% maximum heart rate.
Duration: 45 to 60 minutes.

Resistance training recommendations

Perform one set of eight to 12 repetitions of eight to 10 exercises that condition the major muscle groups at least two days a week minimum.

Tips to keep you exercising

Stay close. Wherever you choose to exercise (gym, park, pool), it should be **no more than 20 minutes away from your home or work**. If you have to travel far to a place to exercise, you run the risk of not wanting to travel, and thus, not wanting to exercise. If it's convenient, it's easier to maintain.

Start an exercise journal or incorporate the information into your food diary (explained in Chapter 4, Step #2). You will be able to see progress. You will also be able to trace back situations when the exercise helped lower your blood sugars.

Have a Plan B. Have some indoor options for exercise planned just in case. During the winter it might be too cold to exercise outdoors, or it might get dark sooner and you are concerned about safety. Or maybe you'll get stuck in traffic and won't get home in time to make your exercise class. Have a Plan B. Ride your stationary bike or play one of your exercise videos instead.

Plan variety into your exercise schedule. If you go to a dance class two times a week, you might want to add a walking workout a couple times a week. I have three different types of exercise I do in any week (what can I say, I get bored easily). I go to Jazzercise two to three times a week and fill the rest of my week in with walks around the neighborhood and evening rides on my stationary bike (while I watch my favorite nighttime television shows).

Make different types of activity part of your normal day. Walking the dog, walking to the mailbox, taking a flight of stairs, walking during part of your lunchbreak are all forms of exercise.

"Check in" with a personal trainer every three months. They can give you specific things you can do, given your personal experiences and preferences. A "check in" session will run you about $30 to $100. Call the American College of Sports Medicine for a list of personal trainers in your area (317-637-9200).

Try something new to keep yourself from getting bored. You could sign up for a class at your local parks and recreation program or through a community college.

You could try a country western dance class, then try yoga, water aerobics, or t'ai chi. Mix it up!

Choose exercise that you actually enjoy. Of course it depends on the person but a large majority of people enjoy walking the most. It's easy, free, and requires only a pair of comfortable shoes. Look around your home or work for lakes or parks that you can walk around after dinner, during the lunch hour, or on the weekends.

4 reasons why people don't exercise

1. It isn't fun!

It isn't exercise per se that isn't fun; it's the *type* of exercise that you have been doing (or not doing) that you are not finding fun. Think about all the possible types of exercise and write down which ones you might find the most fun. Also think about what types of exercise you don't like—and try to put your finger on why you might not be finding it fun. This will give you some clues about what your "fun" exercise options might require.

If you dislike the types of exercise that you do alone, then perhaps you would like exercise that is done as group or team. If you don't think exercising at home is fun, then you should think about exercise that you can do somewhere close to your home—pool aerobics, walking with a buddy, country western dance lessons, etc...

2. There's just no time!

We make time for the things we really *want* to do don't we? And we make time for the things we really *have* to do too. If exercising makes us feel better (and we make it fun) then hopefully it will become something we really *want* to do. If exercising helps us control our blood sugar and body weight (and it does!) then it is also something we really *have* to do—for our health.

Keep in mind that even fitting in 10 minutes of exercise here and there, during the day, can help your body manage diabetes. Walking after a meal or snack (or during a time when your blood sugar tends to be too high) can be particularly helpful for diabetics. The exercise acts like insulin in the body, helping move and use the blood sugar in your blood stream. This doesn't have to be jogging or swimming right after a meal. It could be a quick 10 minute jaunt around your office building after lunch, taking the stairs, walking the dog after dinner, and such.

Instead of "just whistle while you work" how about "just walk while you work." Think about conversations or informal meetings that you can conduct on foot. Take your brainstorming session to the streets. You'd be surprised what some fresh air will do for your creativity. If you are visiting with a neighbor or a if friend pops in for a visit, suggest that you take a walk around your neighborhood while you catch up.

3. It's boring!

Some people get bored more easily than others do. I know—I'm one of them. You may be someone who needs to plan variety into your exercise program. You might want to join a class or league (dance, Jazzercise, water aerobics, swimming, golf, basketball, or tennis) that meets two or three days a week, then fill in the other days with walks, weight training, rowing machine, stationary bicycling, stair climbing, etc. Take lessons for a sport you find interesting.

For many of us, exercising at home on a machine is most convenient. There is no commute time involved. You don't need to find a baby sitter, and it doesn't matter if it rains; once you pay for the machine you exercise for free. If you workout for 30 minutes then it takes exactly 30 minutes out of your day. Us productive types love this! The problem is, this can get a little boring. You ride your bike and row your stationary boat—but you don't actually go anywhere. There's nothing but the wall in front of you to look at. Or is there?

I ride my stationary bike (some of you might find an incumbent bike more comfortable) while I watch a television movie or program that I'm dying to watch. I even fast forward through the commercials if I'm watching a tape. The television keeps my interest while my body is doing the work. If I'm watching something really interesting, the 30 minutes seems to fly by. My husband exercises on his rowing machine while listening to his favorite radio station (something he doesn't get to do very often). You may want to listen to some of your favorite CDs or maybe even a "book on tape."

4. It's raining; it's pouring!

Having several types of exercise options available to you not only adds variety (and minimizes boredom), it gives you an automatic "bad weather" plan. If you have home exercise equipment, you can use it when the weather is cold or wet. If you have signed up for exercise classes or a sports league, they are usually indoors, so you know you will at least get some exercise on those days each week.

If you like to walk and have a walking buddy depending on you, you could very well decide to walk rain or shine. As long as it isn't raining too hard, my walking buddy and I just put our hooded ski jackets on and brave the drops. I find it invigorating! And the warm shower afterwards is truly therapeutic. For more information on exercise and fitness, check out *Fit Happens* by Joanie Greggains, available January 2000 from Villard Publishing.

These are your 10 food steps to freedom. If it seems like too many changes all at once, remember that you can always take it one step at a time.

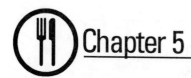 Chapter 5

The 20 Recipes You Can't Live Without

This chapter contains the recipes that will help you follow the 10 food steps to freedom—from eating more omega-3 fatty acids to increasing soluble fiber. Now, I'm sure you've tasted your share of "it's good for you" foods that had absolutely no flavor. Trust me—these recipes don't taste like they're good for you. They just taste great!

Note: The following is a key to the abbreviations used in the recipes: tablespoon (tbs.); teaspoon (tsp.); grams (g); milligrams (mg); Daily Value (DV).

Breakfast Ideas

 ## Light Denver Omelet

I know this looks like it takes a bit of time, but once you know what you're doing, you can whip this out in 10 minutes. If you don't want to whip the egg whites, just beat them into the rest of the egg mixture (it won't be as fluffy, but it still tastes great). This recipe makes 2 servings.

* canola cooking spray
* 1 cup sliced fresh mushrooms (or other vegetable)
* 1 medium green pepper, chopped
* 4 green onions, sliced diagonally
* ¼ tsp. dried basil
* ½ cup chicken broth (water can also be used)
* 3 ounces (½ cup slightly heaping) lean ham, cut into 2-inch long strips
* ½ cup cherry tomatoes, halved (or other tomatoes)
* ½ cup egg substitute
* 2 eggs, separated

1. Coat a medium nonstick frying pan with canola cooking spray, and heat over medium heat. Add mushrooms, green pepper, green onions, and basil. Saute about 30 seconds, then pour in the chicken broth (or water) and cook, stirring frequently, until tender. Stir in ham and cherry tomatoes and cook about a minute to heat through.

2. Blend egg substutute and egg yolks in medium-sized bowl, set aside. With mixer, beat egg whites until stiff. Fold egg whites into egg-yolk mixture.

3. Coat a nonstick omelet or small nonstick frying pan with canola cooking spray (or use 1/2 teaspoon canola oil or canola margarine), and heat over medium-low heat. Spread half of egg mixture in pan. Heat until top looks firm (about 2 minutes). If your pan cooks hotter than normal, cook over low heat. Flip omelet over to lightly brown other side (about 1 minute).

4. Fill with vegetable-ham filling and fold as desired. Remove to serving plate. Repeat with remaining egg mixture to make two fluffy omelets.

Per serving: 190 calories, 9 g carbohydrate, 22 g protein, 7 g fat, 2 g saturated fat, 229 mg cholesterol, 2 g fiber, 690 mg sodium. Calories from fat: 35 percent.

 ## Egg Muffin Sandwich Lite

This recipe makes 2 sandwiches.

- canola cooking spray
- 2 English muffins, toasted
- 1 egg
- ¼ cup egg substitute
- 2 slices Canadian bacon (or thick slices lean ham)
- 1 (6 1/2-oz) empty tuna can (or similar), washed, label removed
- freshly ground pepper
- 2 slices $^{1}/_{3}$ low fat American cheese slices

1. Coat half of a 9-inch nonstick frying pan with canola cooking spray and heat over medium heat.

2. In small bowl, beat the egg with egg substitute; set aside.
3. Place Canadian bacon in the pan over the spray coated area. Spray inside of tuna can with canola cooking spray, and set can on the other side of the pan to start heating. When bottom side of the bacon is light brown, flip over to the other side and cook until light brown. Remove slices from pan and set aside.
4. Pour half of egg mixture (¼ cup) into tuna can. Sprinkle with freshly ground pepper to taste. When the surface of egg begins to firm, cut around the inside of the can with a butter knife to free the edges. Turn the egg over with a cake fork and cook 1 minute more.
5. Remove egg from can.
6. Coat can with canola cooking spray. Repeat with remaining egg.
7. To assemble, layer English muffin bottom with a slice of cheese, then egg, a piece of Canadian bacon, and the English muffin top. To reheat, microwave each sandwich for 20 seconds on high.

Per serving: 287 calories, 21.5 g protein, 30.5 g carbohydrate, 9 g fat, 3.8 g saturated fat, 130 mg cholesterol, 1.5 g fiber, 1100 mg sodium. Calories from fat: 28 percent.

 ## Sun-Dried Tomato-Pesto Spread

Makes spread for about 3 bagels.

- ½ cup light cream cheese
- 1 clove garlic, minced or pressed

- 2 tsp. basil leaves, bottled in water, fresh/chopped, or dried soaked in warm water
- 2 tbs. julienne-style sun-dried tomatoes from bag, soaked in warm water until tender, then drained
- pine nuts, pecans, or walnuts

Add all ingredients to small food processor and process until well blended. Spread on bagels!

Per serving: (with plain bagel) 300 calories, 40.5 g carbohydrate, 14 g protein, 9 g fat, 4.5 g saturated fat, 20 mg cholesterol, 1 g fiber*, 205 mg sodium. Calories from fat: 27 percent.

(*Using a whole grain bagel will add 3 g of fiber per serving.)

 ## The Lox-Ness Monster Spread

Makes about ½ cup of spread (enough for 4 bagels).

- ½ cup light cream cheese
- 2 ounces lox, finely chopped
- 1 green onion, finely chopped
- pinch of fresh or dried dill (optional)
- pinch of capers (optional)

Blend all ingredients in food processor until well mixed. You should still be able to see some small pieces of lox. Spread on bagels.

Per serving: (including plain bagel) 270 calories, 13 g protein, 38.5 g carbohydrate, 7 g fat, 3.5 g saturated fat, 18 mg cholesterol, 1 g fiber*, 560 mg sodium. Calories from fat: 23 percent.

(*Using a whole grain bagel will add 3 g of fiber per serving.)

Apple Lover's Oatmeal

Makes 1 serving.

* 1 packet instant oatmeal, plain (If you use flavored, sweetened instant oatmeal, such as "maple & brown sugar," then don't add the brown sugar.)
* $^1/_3$ cup (or 1 individual serving cup) applesauce, unsweetened
* 2 tbs. brown sugar
* ¼ tsp. ground cinnamon
* ½ cup low-fat milk (or similar—soy milk or almond milk can also be used)

In a large microwave-safe soup bowl, blend all ingredients together. Microwave on high for 1½ minutes. Stir, then microwave for another 1½ minutes. Serve hot.

Per serving: 225 calories, 5.5 g protein, 47 g carbohydrate, 2 grams fat, .8 g saturated fat, 5 mg cholesterol, 2.5 g fiber, 140 mg sodium. Calories from fat: 8 percent.

Note: To make a more balanced breakfast, enjoy this oatmeal with a strip or two of Louis Rich Turkey Bacon.

Flaxseed Recipes

 ## Honey Wheat Bread with Flaxseed

I must have experimented with a dozen different bread machine wheat bread recipes and none were great enough for this book—that is, until I found this one! (For two-pound bread machines.) Makes 12 slices.

- $1^1/_8$ cups water
- 2 ½ cups white bread flour
- ½ cup whole wheat flour
- 1½ tbs.dry milk
- 1 ½ tbs. honey
- 1 ½ tsp. salt
- 2 tbs. canola oil
- ¼ cup ground flaxseed
- 3 tsp. active dry yeast (or 2 tsp. fast-rise yeast)

1. Measure your ingredients and one after the other, load them into your bread machine pan. Add them in the order suggested in your machine owner's manual. (Usually you add the liquids first and end with the dry ingredients. Make a well in your flour and add the yeast.)

2. Adjust the setting for "wheat bread" and then press "Start." This recipe can also be made with rapid or delayed time bake cycles.

3. Let the bread cool slightly before removing from the pan. Use a serrated knife to cut into about 12 slices. Enjoy this bread with canola margarine, reduced fat peanut butter, your favorite preserves, or make your favorite sandwich.

Per serving: 150 calories, 5 g protein, 25 g carbohydrate, 3.8 g fat, 0.5 g saturated fat, 1 mg cholesterol, 2 g fiber, 280 mg sodium. Calories from fat: 19 percent. 0.5 g omega-3 fatty acid per slice (1 g per sandwich).

Flaxseed-Jam Muffins

Makes 9 regular sized muffins.

- $\frac{1}{8}$ cup light or nonfat sour cream
- $\frac{1}{8}$ cup canola oil
- ½ cup low fat milk
- ¼ cup egg substitute (or 1 egg)
- 2 tbs. light corn syrup
- 1 tsp. vanilla extract
- $\frac{2}{3}$ cup unbleached flour
- $\frac{2}{3}$ cup whole wheat flour
- $\frac{1}{3}$ cup ground flaxseed
- ½ cup granulated sugar
- 2 tsp. baking powder
- ½ tsp. salt
- about 4 tbs. jam of your choice

1. Preheat oven to 375 degrees. Coat 9 muffin cups with canola cooking spray.
2. Place sour cream in a glass mixing bowl. Warm briefly in the microwave so it will blend easier. Stir in oil and milk, a tablespoon at a time. Stir in egg or egg substitute, corn syrup, and vanilla extract.
3. Blend flours, flaxseed, sugar, baking powder, salt together and add all at once to liquid mixture. Stir just enough to moisten.
4. Fill each mini muffin cup with a level ¼ cup measure of batter. Spoon about 1½ teaspoons jam in the center of each muffin.

5. Bake about 18 to 20 minutes for regular sized muffins or until golden brown and muffin tests done.

Per serving: (using reduced sugar jam) 197 calories, 4.5 g protein, 35.5 g carbohydrate, 5 g fat, 0.5 g saturated fat, 1 mg cholesterol, 3 g fiber, 260 mg sodium. Calories from fat: 23 percent. 1.5 g omega-3 fatty acids.

 ## Flaxseed Focaccia

This recipe calls for fresh rosemary (or dried) in the dough. If you don't care for rosemary just leave it out. You probably won't notice the flaxseed in this bread—it is fragrant, moist, and delicious! Cut the focaccia into servings and freeze in a Ziplock bag. Then when you need some, just thaw a serving or two in the microwave. (This recipe is for bread machines.)

Makes 8 servings (Each serving will make a sandwich.).

Dough:

- $1^{1}/_{3}$ cups water
- 1 tbs. finely chopped fresh rosemary leaves or 1½ teaspoon dried rosemary leaves
- 2 tsp. salt
- 3 tbs. olive oil
- ½ cup cornmeal
- 2¾ cups unbleached white flour
- $^{1}/_{3}$ cup ground flaxseed
- 1 packet (3 tsp.) fast-acting yeast

Topping:

- 3 tbs. olive oil
- 1 tbs. chopped or minced garlic

- 1 tbs. finely chopped fresh basil leaves
- ¼ tsp. salt (optional)
- ¼ cup shredded parmesan cheese

1. Add all the dough ingredients, in this order, into the bread machine pan. Set for "dough" and press "Start." Check dough after five minutes and add water, a teaspoon at a time if necessary, to make a smooth, soft ball of dough.

2. In the meantime, add 3 tablespoons olive oil, garlic, basil leaves and ½ teaspoon salt if desired to a small bowl. Blend ingredients and let sit on counter until needed.

3. When dough is ready (after about 1 hour 40 minutes) preheat oven to 425 degrees and make sure the oven rack is in the center position. Sprinkle a heavy baking sheet with extra cornmeal.

4. Remove the dough from the machine to a lightly floured work surface. Pat dough into a 1-inch thick round or square. Place it on the prepared baking sheet and poke dimples all over the surface of the dough with your fingertips. Cover with a clean towel and allow to rise on or near oven as it warms up for about 30 minutes.

5. Spread the oil mixture over the top and sprinkle with shredded parmesan cheese.

6. Bake focaccia for 10 minutes then reduce heat to 350 degrees. Bake about 10 to 12 minutes more, or until top is golden.

7. Use as a side dish or for a gourmet sandwich.

Per serving: 314 calories, 8 g protein, 42.5 g carbohydrate, 12 g fat, 2 g saturated fat, 2 mg cholesterol, 3 g fiber, 593 mg sodium. Calories from fat: 35 percent. 1.7 g omega-3 fatty acids.

Flaxseed Maple Scones

If you even barely like the taste of maple, you will find these scones addicting! I even converted the recipe to a food processor to make these scones a cinch to make. These scones are loaded with ground flaxseed so one scone will give you a day's supply of flaxseed. They freeze well in Ziplock bags. You can even eat them right out of the freezer! This recipe makes 8 scones.

- canola cooking spray
- 1½ cups all purpose flour
- $\frac{1}{3}$ cup oats
- ½ cup ground flaxseed
- 2 tbs. sugar
- ½ tsp. salt
- 1 tbs. baking powder
- 2 tbs. maple syrup
- 2 tbs. canola oil
- 1 egg
- ½ cup whole milk (lowfat milk will work too)
- ½ tsp. maple extract (¾ teaspoon if you want a stronger maple flavor in the dough)
- $\frac{2}{3}$ cup coarsely chopped pecans (a little smaller than "pecan pieces" but bigger than "finely chopped pecans)

Maple glaze:

- 1½ cups powdered sugar
- ½ tsp. maple extract
- 5 tsp. water

1. Preheat oven to 425 degrees. Make an 8-inch circle with canola cooking spray on a thick baking sheet.

2. Add flour, oats, flaxseed, sugar, salt, and baking powder to food processor bowl. Pulse to mix and finely grind the oats with the flour.

3. Add maple syrup and canola oil to the flour mixture and pulse to blend the two well.

4. In a separate small bowl, beat the egg lightly with the milk and 1/2 teaspoon maple extract. Pour the milk mixture into the flour mixture in the food processor. Pulse briefly to make a dough.

5. Place dough on well floured surface. Sprinkle pecans over the top and knead lightly four times to evenly distribute the pecans. Pat dough into a 7½-inch circle. Cut into 8 wedges. Place wedges in a circle on prepared baking sheet. Bake in center of oven for about 13 to 15 minutes (top will be lightly browned).

6. While scones are baking, combine glaze ingredients to a small bowl and stir well until smooth. Remove scones from oven to wire rack and let cool about three to five minutes. Spread glaze generously over each scone. Once glaze has dried (about 15 minutes) the scones can be served! They keep well overnight in a Ziplock bag.

Per serving: 330 calories, 6 g protein, 51 g carbohydrate, 12 g fat, 4 g fiber, 38 mg cholesterol, 370 mg sodium. Calories from fat: 33 percent. 1.3 g omega-3 fatty acids.

Note: Because the fat grams come mainly from the pecans and the canola oil, most of the fat is the preferred monounsaturated fat!

Best Bean Recipes

 ## High Legume Fried Rice

Makes 4 servings.

- 3 tbs. canola oil
- ¼ cup sliced green onions, packed
- ¾ cup frozen green peas
- ¾ cup boiled or canned soy beans (Some super-markets carry "boiled soy beans in pod" in the freezer section.) If using frozen follow the d i - rections on the bag to finish cooking it then re-move the soy beans from the pods.
- ½ cup diced lean ham (optional)
- 4 cups cooked steamed rice
- 1 egg beaten with ¼ cup egg substitute
- ½ tsp. salt
- 1 to 2 tbs. light or regular soy sauce

1. Heat oil in wok or large nonstick saucepan to very hot. Add green onion and let sit for one minute.
2. Add green peas, soy beans, ham if desired, and rice and let sit for a minute.
3. Push away the mixture toward the edges of the pan, leaving the middle of pan open, and pour in the egg mixture.
4. Let sit for about 20 seconds then begin to stir the eggs for another 20 seconds.
5. Stir-fry the entire mixture together for a couple of minutes, sprinkling salt and soy sauce over the top. Add more soy sauce at table if desired.

Per serving: (with 2 tablespoons light soy sauce) 448 calories, 14.5 g protein, 64 g carbohydrate, 14 g fat, 1.5 g saturated fat, 53 mg cholesterol, 6 g fiber, 590 mg sodium. Calories from fat: 28 percent.

 ## 3-Minute Burrito

Makes 1 burrito.

- ½ cup cooked or canned pinto beans or pinquitos (small brown beans), drained and rinsed
- 1 tbs. chopped fresh cilantro (optional)
- 2 tbs. light or fat free sour cream
- 1 green onion, chopped
- $\frac{1}{8}$ cup chunky salsa (mild or hot depending on preference)
- 1 burrito size flour tortilla
- 1½ ounces reduced-fat Monterey jack or sharp cheddar cheese, grated (about a heaping $\frac{1}{3}$ cup)

1. In small bowl, toss beans, cilantro if desired, sour cream, green onion, and salsa together.
2. Heat tortilla in microwave on a double thickness of paper towel for about 1 minute or until soft.
3. Sprinkle cheese evenly over the tortilla.
4. Spread bean mixture in center of tortilla. Fold bottom and top ends of tortilla in and roll up into a burrito.
5. Microwave one more minute or until burrito is heated through.

Per serving: 430 calories, 23.5 g protein, 53.5 g carbohydrate, 14.5 g fat, 7 grams saturated fat, 26 mg cholesterol, 6 g fiber, 480 mg sodium. Calories from fat: 30 percent.

Pintos and Cheese

Makes 1 serving.

- ½ cup fat-free or vegetarian refried beans
- 2 tbs. salsa (or 1 tsp. chili sauce), or to taste
- 1 ounce reduced-fat Monterey Jack cheese, grated

1. Spread half of beans in microwave-safe serving bowl. Top beans with half of the salsa.
2. In small bowl, toss grated cheese with green onion. Sprinkle half of cheese and onion mixture over beans.
3. Spread remaining beans over the top then add remaining salsa.
4. Sprinkle remaining cheese and onion over the top.
5. Microwave on high for 2 to 3 minutes or until cheese bubbles.

Per serving: 215 calories, 12 g protein, 29.5 g carbohydrate, 6 g fat, 3 g saturated fat, 15 mg cholesterol, 7 g fiber, 750 mg sodium. Calories from fat: 25 percent.

 ## Quick-Fix Chili and Fries

Makes 2 servings.

- 12 ounces lowfat frozen french fries (OreIda Country Fries or Steak Fries)
- 2 ounces reduced fat sharp cheddar, grated (about ½ cup firmly packed)
- 15 ounces vegetarian canned chili (Hormel brand works well)

1. Preheat oven to 450 degrees. Arrange frozen French fries in a single layer on baking sheet or shallow pan. Bake 20 to 25 minutes, turning after 15 minutes, or until desired crispness and color.
2. Spoon chili into two serving bowls. Heat in microwave (about 3 minutes for each bowl on high) or place in a small casserole dish; heat in oven along with the French fries.
3. Sprinkle grated cheese over the chili before serving. Serve with fries on the side.

Per serving: 500 calories, 25 g protein, 77 g carbohydrate, 10 g fat, 3 g saturated fat, 20 mg cholesterol, 13 g fiber, 1080 mg sodium. Calories from fat: 18 percent.

Quick Omega-3 Entrees

 ## Lemon Dijon Salmon

Makes 2 servings.

- canola cooking spray
- 2 salmon steaks (about 6 ounces each)
- 1 tbs. Dijon mustard
- garlic salt (about ½ tsp.)
- freshly ground pepper
- ½ onion, thinly sliced
- ½ lemon
- about 2 to 3 tsp. capers

1. Preheat oven to 400 degrees. Line a 9-inch pie plate with a large sheet of foil (enough so it can

be wrapped back over the fish and sealed) and spray foil generously with canola cooking spray. Lay salmon steaks in prepared pan.

2. Spread fish steaks evenly with Dijon mustard.

3. Sprinkle fish steaks with garlic salt and ground pepper to your liking.

4. Lay thinly sliced onion over the top.

5. Squeeze lemon over the top of the salmon and sprinkle capers over the top.

6. Wrap edges of foil over the top of fish and seal edges together. Bake about 15 minutes. Open foil and let bake about 5 minutes more or until salmon is cooked throughout.

7. Serve with steamed rice or cooked pasta and some vegetables.

Per serving: 231 calories, 30 g protein, 5 g carbohydrate, 10 g fat, 1.5 g saturated fat, 80 mg cholesterol, 1 g fiber, 678 mg sodium. Calories from fat: 39 percent.

Per serving: (when each serving is served with ¾ cup steamed rice and a cup of broccoli) 475 calories, 38.5 g protein, 56 g carbohydrate, 11 g fat, 1.7 g saturated fat, 80 mg cholesterol, 6.5 g fiber, 720 mg sodium. Calories from fat: 21 percent. 5.5 grams omega-3 fatty acids.

 ## Simple Salmon Pasta Salad

This is one of my favorite salads. I make extra grilled salmon on purpose so I can make this salad the next day with the leftovers. This recipe makes about 2 entrée servings.

- 3 cups bow tie or rotelle pasta made with semolina flour, cooked al dente

- 1 cup salmon flakes (freshly cooked or grilled salmon fillets or steaks, broken into flakes with fork, with no bones or skin)
- 1 cup crisp-tender asparagus pieces, steamed or microwaved
- 3 green onions, finely chopped

Dressing:

- 1 tbs. canola mayonnaise (if available otherwise use regular)
- 3 tbs. fat-free or light sour cream
- 1 tbs. lemon juice
- 1½ tsp. Dijon or prepared mustard
- ½ tsp. dill weed
- black pepper to taste

1. Place pasta, salmon, asparagus and green onions in serving bowl.
2. Blend dressing ingredients in a 1- or 2-cup measure until smooth. Add to pasta salad ingredients and stir to mix.

Per serving: 339 calories, 18 g protein, 45 g carbohydrate, 9.5 g fat, 1.5 g saturated fat, 29 mg cholesterol, 3 g fiber, 122 mg sodium. Calories from fat: 26 percent. 1 g omega-3 fatty acid per serving.

 ## Easy Omega-3 Fatty Acid Tuna Sandwich

Makes 2 sandwiches.

- 6½ ounces albacore tuna, drained
- 1 tbs. sweet or dill pickle relish (optional)

- ¼ tsp. salt (optional)
- 1 tbs.canola mayonnaise (or regular)
- ½ tbs.minced onion
- ¼ cup minced celery
- 1 tbs.light or fat-free sour cream
- pepper to taste
- 2 slices whole wheat or whole grain bread
- lettuce leaves and tomato slices

1. Add tuna, relish, salt, mayo, sour cream, onion, and celery together in small bowl; mix well. Add pepper to taste.
2. Spread mixture on slices of bread to make a sandwich. Add lettuce leaves, and tomato slices.

Per serving: 320 calories, 27 g protein, 34 g carbohydrate, 10 g fat, 1.4 g saturated fat, 27 mg cholesterol, 4.5 g fiber, 676 mg sodium. Calories from fat: 25 percent. About 0.5 g omega-3 fatty acids from tuna and about 0.5 from the canola mayonnaise.

Other Quick Entrées

 Oat Bran Meat Loaf

This meat loaf tastes so much better than it sounds. Each serving contributes 5 grams of mostly soluble fiber to the meal too! This recipe makes 5 servings.

- canola cooking spray
- 1¼ canned chick-peas (garbanzo beans), drained and rinsed

- ½ cup oat bran
- ½ tsp. black pepper
- ½ tsp. salt (optional)
- 2 cloves garlic, minced or pressed, or ½ tsp. garlic powder
- 1 tbs. Worcestershire sauce
- 2 tbs. Heinz chili sauce
- 1 tbs. prepared mustard
- 1 pound ground sirloin (about 9 percent fat)
- 1 cup grated reduced fat sharp cheddar cheese (optional)
- 1 small onion, finely chopped
- 1 cup tomato sauce

1. Preheat oven to 350 degrees. Coat a 9-by-5-inch loaf pan with canola cooking spray.
2. Add all ingredients up to and including mustard to mixer or food processor. You can also mash with pastry blender or potato masher.
3. Process until well mixed (there will be some lumps).
4. If using a mixer, add beef, cheese, and onion to bean mixture and mix until well blended. If using a food processor, blend bean mixture with beef, cheese, and onion with hands (or use a spoon) in a large mixing bowl.
5. Add mixture to pan and form into a loaf.
6. Bake 30 minutes. Pour tomato sauce over the top and bake 15 minutes longer.

Per serving: 286 calories, 24.5 g protein, 28.5 g carbohydrate, 10 g fat, 3.5 g saturated fat, 33 mg cholesterol, 5 g fiber, 700 mg sodium. Calories from fat: 29 percent.

Light Club Sandwich

This recipe makes 1 sandwich.

* 2 slices Louis Rich turkey bacon (or a similar brand)
* 3 slices whole wheat bread
* 1 teaspoon canola mayonnaise (or regular) blended with 1 teaspoon of light or fat-free sour cream
* 2 lettuce leaves
* 1 large slice turkey breast (about 2 ounces)
* pepper to taste
* $1/_2$ large tomato, sliced

1. Cook bacon in nonstick frying pan over low heat until crisp.
2. Spread one side of each bread slice lightly with mayonnaise mixture. Arrange lettuce leaf on one slice; top with one slice of turkey; sprinkle with pepper, then cover with another bread slice, mayonnaise side up. Top with another leaf of lettuce, tomato slices, bacon slices, and remaining bread slice, mayonnaise side down.
3. Cut the sandwich diagonally into fourths; secure each quarter with decorated toothpicks, if desired.

Per serving: 350 calories, 19 g protein, 38 g carbohydrate, 12.5 g fat, 2.7 g saturated fat, 49 mg cholesterol, 5.5 g fiber, 1400 mg sodium. Calories from fat: 32 percent.

Scrumptious Side Dishes

 ## Monounsaturated Side Salad

This salad is not just rich in monounsaturated fats—it's rich in fiber. This recipe makes 4 servings.

- ½ avocado, cut into bite-size pieces
- ½ cucumber, sliced
- 1 cup chopped tomatoes or cherry tomatoes cut in half
- 1 cup kidney beans (or ½ cup kidney beans and ½ cup garbanzo) drained and rinsed
- 6 tbs. bottled vinaigrette (or other dressing that uses olive oil or canola oil)
- 4 to 6 cups read-to-serve salad greens of your choice

1. Toss avocado, cucumber, tomatoes, and beans into a serving bowl. Toss with dressing; set aside in refrigerator until needed.
2. Right before mealtime, toss vegetable mixture with lettuce.

Per serving: 155 calories, 6 g protein, 19 g carbohydrate, 7 g fat, .7 g saturated fat, 0 mg cholesterol, 7 g fiber, 460 mg sodium. Calories from fat: 43 percent.

 ## Easy 3-Bean Salad

Makes 4 servings.

- 8¾-ounce can kidney beans, drained and rinsed (about 1 cup)

- 8¾-ounce can garbanzo beans, drained and rinsed (about 1 cup)
- 8¾-ounce can green or yellow wax beans, drained and rinsed (about 1 cup)
- ¼ cup finely diced yellow or white onion
- 4 tbs. bottled vinaigrette (that uses olive oil or canola oil)

Combine all ingredients in serving bowl. Toss well. This stores well for several days if covered in the refrigerator.

Per serving: 160 calories, 7 g protein, 27.5 g carbohydrate, 3 g fat, 0 g saturated fat, 0 mg cholesterol, 7 g fiber, 635 mg sodium. Calories from fat: 17 percent.

Quick snacks and pick-me-ups

 ## Quick Ranch Dip (with vegetables)

Makes about ¼ cup of dip.

- 1 tsp. Hidden Valley Ranch Dip powder
- ¼ cup light or nonfat sour cream
- 1 tsp. canola mayonnaise (if available), otherwise, use regular
- assorted raw vegetables for dipping (baby carrots, celery sticks, broccoli, and cauliflower florets)

1. Combine all dip ingredients in a small bowl. Stir well with spoon.
2. Serve with assorted vegetables.

Per serving: ($^1/_8$ cup dip with 1 cup raw vegetables) 95 calories, 3 g protein, 16.5 g carbohydrate, 2 g fat, .2 g saturated fat, 1 mg cholesterol, 3.3 g fiber, 325 mg sodium. Calories from fat: 19 percent.

 ## Spicy Hummus with Crudites and Crackers

This is a variation on the really tasty middle Eastern dip/spread. You may have to search a bit to find tahini, although it is available in many supermarkets on the East and West Coasts. This recipe makes about 3 cups of dip.

- 15½-ounce can 50% less-sodium garbanzo beans
- 3 cloves garlic, minced or pressed
- $^1/_3$ cup tahini (sesame seed paste)
- ¼ cup lemon juice
- 3 tbs. light or fat free sour cream
- 2 tbs. light cream cheese
- ¼ tsp. seasoning salt (optional)
- ¼ tsp. ground cumin
- ¼ tsp. paprika
- 2 tbs. finely chopped fresh parsley (optional)
- crudites: choose crisp vegetables like red bell pepper, carrots, celery, cauliflower, broccoli, green beans, etc.
- crackers: choose from many reduced-fat crackers on the market

1. Drain garbanzo beans and rinse well. (Reserve some of the liquid to add back if you need it to make a thinner dip.)

2. Place beans, garlic, tahini, lemon juice, sour cream, cream cheese, seasoning salt if desired, cumin, paprika, and parsley in food processor. Blend until somewhat smooth. Add more lemon juice or garbanzo liquid to taste. Use immediately or cover and refrigerate (will keep for several days). Serve with vegetables and crackers.

Per serving: ($^1/_3$ cup dip) 100 calories, 1 g protein, 9 g carbohydrate, 5.5 g fat, 1 g saturated fat, 1 mg cholesterol, 3 g fiber*, 120 mg sodium. Calories from fat: 50 percent.

*When each serving is eaten with a cup of suggested vegetables the fiber increases to about 6 g a serving.

 ## Iced Café Mocha

This is a great drink to slip two teaspoons of ground flaxseed into. If you want to use the reduced-sugar chocolate syrup, go ahead, but I personally don't care for the flavor. This recipe makes 1 drink.

- 4 ice cubes
- 2 level tsp. instant espresso powder (available in coffee section of most supermarkets)
- 1 cup 1% or 2% lowfat milk
- 2 tbs. chocolate syrup

1. Place ice cubes in blender or food processor and pulse until crushed.
2. In small cup blend espresso powder with 2 tablespoons of the milk.
3. Add to blender along with remaining milk and chocolate syrup. Pulse until nicely blended. Pour into cup and enjoy!

Per serving: 185 calories, 9 g protein, 31 g carbohydrate, 3 g fat, 1.6 g saturated fat, 10 mg cholesterol, 1 g fiber, 165 mg sodium. Calories from fat: 15 percent.

 ## Oatmeal Raisin Bites

You can make a batch of these babies then pop them in the freezer in a Ziplock bag. Take out a cookie whenever you need it, it thaws quickly in the microwave or at room temperature. This recipe makes 32 large cookies.

- 6 tbs. canola margarine or butter, softened
- 6 tbs. fat-free or light cream cheese
- 1 cup packed brown sugar
- ½ cup granulated sugar
- ¼ cup low-fat buttermilk
- ¼ cup egg substitute
- 2 tbs. maple syrup
- 2 tsp. vanilla extract
- 1 cup unbleached flour
- ½ tsp. baking soda
- 1½ tsp. ground cinnamon
- ¼ tsp. salt
- 3 cups quick or old fashioned oats
- 1 cup raisins
- ½ cup chopped walnuts (optional)

1. Preheat oven to 350 degrees. Coat two cookie sheets with canola cooking spray. In a large bowl, beat the butter with cream cheese. Beat

in the sugars, buttermilk, egg substitute, maple syrup, and vanilla and beat until light and fluffy.

2. Combine the flour, baking soda, cinnamon, and salt; beat into the butter mixture, mixing well.

3. Stir in the oats, raisins, and nuts if desired, mixing well.

4. Use a cookie scoop (or drop by rounded table-spoonfuls) to form cookies and place 2 inches apart on the prepared cookie sheets. For flatter rather than rounded cookies, press each cookie mound down lightly with a spoon, spatula, or your fingers.

5. Bake one cookie sheet at a time, in the upper third of oven for about 10 minutes, or until lightly browned. Remove the cookies to wire racks to cool completely. Store in an airtight container.

Per serving: 120 calories, 2 g protein, 22 g carbohydrate, 3 g fat, .4 g saturated fat, 5 mg cholesterol, 1.2 g fiber, 36 mg sodium. Calories from fat: 22 percent.

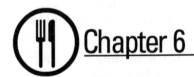

Chapter 6

Navigating the Supermarket

It's easy to get confused while shopping in the trenches (a.k.a. your typical grocery store). Each product label your eye catches inevitably hits you with countless advertising slogans and nutrition terms. Just remember the bottom line is that all these companies are basically trying to sell you something—they all want a piece of your food budget. The package might boast "sugar free" or "fat free" but it's the nutrition information label that's going to tell you whether that product has just as many grams of carbohydrate or just as many calories as the regular products.

It's also the nutrition information label that is going to confess what the company thinks the serving size is. A single serving of a Snickers candy bar is about half of a 2-ounce bar. A serving of most ice creams is usually a half cup. A serving of some of the cookie brands is one cookie while the serving of many pot pies is half a pot pie. The serving size of many individual or small-sized frozen pizzas is one-third of the "small" pizza. There is some "reduced fat" ice cream bars out there that, when you check the label, still contain over 13 grams of fat per serving. The moral of this story is—read your labels. The more you know about the product, the better off you will be.

How to speak supermarket-ese

Here are the definitions of some of the labeling or advertising terms that you might be most interested in:

Free means that a product contains no or only negligible amounts of some percentage of fat, saturated fat, cholesterol, sodium, sugar, and/or calories.

"% fat free" is used only on low-fat or fat-free products. The term is a reflection of the amount of the food's weight that is fat free. For example, if a serving of food weighs 100 grams and two of the grams come from fat, it can be called "98 percent fat free."

"Low" means different things in different circumstances:

- Low calorie: 40 calories or less per serving.

- Low fat: 3 grams or fewer per serving.

- Low saturated fats: no more than 1 gram per serving.

- Low cholesterol: fewer than 20 milligrams per serving.

- Low sodium: fewer than 140 milligrams per serving.

"Reduced" lets the customer know that a product has been nutritionally altered and contains 25 percent less of a nutrient or of calories than the regular product.

"Light" means the product contains 50 percent less fat (in grams) than the regular product or the calories have been reduced by at least one-third of what they were in the regular product. *"Light"* can also be used to refer to the texture and color of a food; however, the label must spell this out (for example, light brown sugar).

"Daily values" on the new nutrition labels means how a food fits into the overall daily diet. The daily values are based on a daily diet of 2,000 calories (individuals are supposed to adjust the values to fit their own calorie intake). The daily values provide figures for fat, saturated fat, cholesterol, sodium, carbohydrates, fiber, vitamins and minerals.

A sugar by any other name

Sugars or sweeteners can go by many names other than "sugar." Other names for sugar that you might see on an ingredient label are:

- Sucrose.
- High fructose corn syrup.
- Fructose.
- Brown sugar.
- Maltose.
- Corn sweeteners.
- Dextrose.
- Honey.
- Syrups (such as corn syrup, maple syrup or molasses).

Don't let all this confuse you too much. You'll get the information you need for your counting and calculating from the nutrition information label—grams of total carbohydrate per serving. (Make sure and check out the serving size—it might surprise you.)

Supermarket 101

There are several lessons to be learned before navigating the supermarket— with or without diabetes. The first is to *look to the label*—check the portion size, the grams of fat, carbohydrates, and calories when shopping for and comparing food products.

The second lesson is a bit more difficult to master. Some of us may be using these fat-free products as an excuse to overeat. I don't think we are entirely to blame here. If these products aren't as satisfying, we're probably more likely to keep on eating and eating in the hope of reaching some level of satisfaction. Also, some of the advertising has basically encouraged us to eat as much as we want—after all, it's fat-free! So select only those light and fat-free products that you truly like, that taste satisfying to you, and that you can eat in modest serving sizes. Otherwise, they aren't going to do a hill of beans for your health and enjoyment.

For example, I really love Cracker Barrel Light Sharp Cheddar; it is real cheese to me. My family has Louis Rich turkey bacon, and we don't miss real bacon. Reduced Fat Bisquick is a staple in my house. We all think Louis Rich turkey franks and Ball Park Lite franks taste terrific. These are the types of products you want to keep buying—the ones that you truly enjoy.

Last but not least, figure the grams of carbohydrate into your daily eating plan.

When sampling some of the new fat-free or sugar-free products, you will quickly learn that some companies have definitely gone too far. In my opinion, certain foods simply aren't meant to be fat free. If you take all the fat out of a food that was mostly fat to begin with, such as mayonnaise, cheese, or butter, then what have you really got? Something other than mayonnaise, cheese, or butter—that's for sure. It's not fat-free butter; it's just a new kind of yellow goop.

More than half of the new fat-free, sugar-free, or "light" products I try end up in the garbage can. But the upside is that about 20 percent (or one in five) of the products are keepers. A number of products have successfully hit their optimal level of fat. These are the foods that withstood a modest reduction in fat without a huge loss in taste satisfaction. You'll find them listed in this chapter.

Avoiding the land mines

Have you ever noticed that the Nutrition Facts information on the label of a baking mix or cake mix is listed in two columns: *Mix* and *Baked* (or *As Prepared*)? Normally they will give you two amounts of fat grams: one from the mix and one for the total amount of fat per serving after it is prepared. This is important information, because many of these mixes call for one-third cup of oil, or three eggs, or a stick of butter.

Several companies have started giving only the grams of fat in the mix. If you look real closely, which is what I get paid to do, you'll see a tiny asterisk next to the grams of fat. Then you look down at the very bottom of the label and in small print it reads something like this: "Amount in mix."

They do give you the percent daily value for grams of fat "as prepared," but let's face it, what does that really mean to most people. Most people just quickly scan the label until they see grams of fat. I can just picture people thinking, "Oh, goody, 4 grams of fat!" When in reality, if they follow the directions on the box, a serving has something more like 9 or 13 grams of fat per serving.

Just so you know what to watch out for—here is an example.

Pillsbury Thick 'n Fudgy Cheesecake Swirl Deluxe Brownie Mix: According to the label, a serving of mix contains 4.5 grams of fat. When you follow the directions on the box, adding one-quarter cup oil and two eggs to the mix, the grams of fat per serving increases to 9 grams of fat. But you don't see 9 grams anywhere on the label. If you look real hard you'll find 14 percent daily value for fat in the "prepared" column. You have to do a little math to get to 9 from the 14% Daily Value given on the label.

It's all in a name

We've come to rely on certain brands with diet-sounding names to steer us toward the better choices where our waistlines and diabetes are concerned. Weight Watchers, Lean Cuisine, and Slim Fast, for example, are all music to the ears. Don't let those seductive names fool you. Some of these products are just as high in calories, fat, and carbohydrate grams as the overtly "sinful" products farther down the aisle.

In many cases what they are selling you is portion control and a pretty name (for a handsome price). The Nestle Sweet Success Peanut Butter snack bar weighs in at 31 grams with 100 calories, 3.5 grams of fat and 23 grams of carbohydrate. Now jog just a few feet farther

---

F.Y.I. A little math lesson

If you look at the percent daily value guide at the very bottom of the label (in smaller print), you see "less than 65 grams of fat" listed for a 2,000-calorie standard intake. Now multiply 65 grams by 14 percent and you get 9 grams of fat.

and you'll find Kudos Peanut Butter bar with 130 calories, 5 grams fat and less carbohydrate—19 grams.

But at least it's not like eating a candy bar, right? Wrong. Twenty-eight grams of Milky Way (half of a regular sized bar) actually contains almost the same amount of calories (118) and fat (4 grams) as the Slim Fast and Nestle Sweet Success snack bars.

Fat-free but full of calories

Here's a newsflash—just because a product is fat-free doesn't mean it is calorie-free or that you can eat the whole box in one sitting. In fact, many of these fat-free products have just as many calories as the full-fat versions. How can that be? In a word—sugar. Sugar, whether it comes from honey, corn syrup, brown sugar, or high fructose corn syrup, can add moisture and help tenderize bakery products. When added to foods like ice cream, it adds flavor and structure. So I'm not surprised that manufacturers have turned to sugar for assistance while developing reduced-fat and fat-free products.

The majority of the fat-free and lower-fat products on the supermarket shelves only offer us average savings of 10 or 20 calories per serving. Does this mean we shouldn't buy any of these products? No—this means to truly benefit from these lower-fat or fat-free products, we need to watch our serving size and keep track of the grams of carbohydrates we are taking in.

Taking a tour of your supermarket

I walked around my supermarket, pen and paper in hand, with an eye for foods and products that someone like you might want to know about:

- I looked for lower carbohydrate and reduced calorie products that might come in handy when you are trying to balance a meal or snack.
- I looked for good, easy sources of soluble fiber.
- I looked for quick sources of omega-3 fatty acids and monounsaturated fats.
- I looked for whole grain products that would contribute fiber and other nutrients, and also possibly have a positive effect on our blood sugars.
- I also included nutrition information for convenience products you might be tempted to buy, so you can make the very best choices.

A note before we continue: In the remainder of this chapter and in the chapter that follows, you will find many helpful tables. We have abbreviated some items for space considerations. They are: Cal. (Calories), Carbs. (Carbohydrates), Pro. (Protein), Fib. (Fiber), Sat. (Saturated fat) and Sod. (Sodium). Are you ready? Here we go...

Frozen breakfast foods

You can buy everything from breakfast muffins to a complete egg sausage and hash brown breakfast in the frozen food section. Watch out, though. Frozen breakfast foods are either brimming with saturated or trans fats or sugar. You've got to keep an eye out for flashy health claims, too. There is a popular brand boasting that their "Healthy Muffins" are fiber rich, but you can get just as much fiber (and a lot less sugar) from a bowl of Cheerios. I've listed the frozen waffles that contain some fiber and some lighter frozen sausages that might help balance out an otherwise mostly carbohydrate breakfast, and added a few frozen breakfast convenience products that are fairly well balanced between fat, carbohydrate, and protein.

Frozen Breakfast Foods

	Cal.	Carbs (g)	Fat (g, %*)	Pro. (g)	Fib. (g)	Sod. (mg)
Eggo Golden Oat waffles (made w/ oat bran), 2	140	26	2.5 (16%)	5	3	270
Eggo Raisin & Bran waffles, 2	210	36	6 (26%)	5	5	430
Eggo Nutri-Grain Multigrain waffles, 2	160	29	5 (28%)	5	5	360
Jones Brown & Serve Light (pork and rice links), 2	110	1	9 (73%)	7	0	280
Swift Premium Brown 'N Serve, 3	120	1	9 (67%)	7	0	280
Weight Watchers Smart Ones: English Muffin sandwich	210	28	5 (21%)	13	2	420
Weight Watchers Smart Ones: Handy Ham & Cheese Omelet	320	30	5 (14%)	13	2	440
Amy's Organic Black Bean Ranchero Breakfast Burrito	230	38	5 (19%)	9	5	480

*Percent calories from fat

Do you like hashbrowns?

Like hashbrowns but loathe all the fat the frozen hashbrowns have? There's a frozen hashbrown you can buy that comes with no fat. You can decide how much and which oil to add when you pan fry them. You can fry them in a little bit of canola oil and make a crispy, tasty hashbrown that contributes monounsaturated fat, and some omega-3 fatty acids to boot. Take a look:

OreIda Hash Browns: One patty contains 70 calories, 0 fat and cholesterol, 16 grams carbohydrate, 2 grams protein, 1 gram fiber, and 30 milligrams sodium.

Pan fry three of the patties in one tablespoon of canola oil (fry for about six minutes, turn and fry four minutes more): one patty contains 110 calories, 4.5 grams fat (3 grams of which are monounsaturated), and 36 percent calories from fat.

Egg Substitutes

	Calories	Carbs (g)	Fat (g)	Protein (g)	Sodium (mg)
Egg Beaters	30	1	0	6	125
Scramblers	35	2	0	6	95
All Whites (Papetti Foods)	33	2.5	0	7	100

Egg substitutes

People with Type II diabetes sometimes manage a meal better if it contains *some* fat (instead of no fat or very low fat). So, using egg substitutes (which are both fat- and cholesterol-free) in meals that are fat free may not be the best idea. There are two ways that egg substitutes can be your saving grace:

1. Use egg substitutes in recipes or meals that are high fat to help bring down the total fat to a more moderate level.

2. Use part egg substitutes and part real eggs in baking and cooking to help bring down the cholesterol per serving.

Using egg substitutes increases the protein too because egg substitutes are mostly egg white—the protein portion of the egg. (Remember all the fat and cholesterol is in the yolk of the egg.) My favorite brand of egg substitute (Egg Beaters) is 99 percent egg white, which explains why it has almost no fat and very few calories. It looks like scrambled eggs so you can use it in omelets, quiche, and any recipe that calls for beaten eggs. If you use half egg substitute and half real eggs, you will usually have a food or recipe that tastes very similar to the original. For example, if the recipe calls for four eggs, you could use two eggs and a half-cup egg substitute (one-quarter cup per egg it replaces).

Do you like donuts?

Have you tried the Entenmann's Light donuts yet? Well, you should. Of course, it isn't something you should eat every breakfast. But if you have a hankering for a donut, this will satisfy with 50 percent less fat and a little less calories too. Entenmann's offers two variety packs:

The Light Variety Pack, 1 donut contains: 190 calories, 31 grams carbohydrate, 7 grams fat (33 percent calories from fat), 1.5 grams saturated fat, 3 grams protein, 15 milligrams cholesterol, < 1 gram fiber, and 320 milligrams sodium.

The Light Chocolate Lover's Variety Pack, 1 donut contains: 220 calories, 34 grams carbohydrate, 9 grams fat (37% calories from fat), 2.5 grams saturated fat, 2 grams protein, 15 milligrams cholesterol, <1 gram fiber, and 270 milligrams sodium.

Diabetic-friendly frozen entrees

Frozen entrees come in handy in many situations—as a quick lunch during the workweek and as an easy dinner if you live alone or with one other person.

The problem with frozen entrees is that the ones that are lower in fat are almost always too low in calories and carbohydrate and meager in the vegetable department. They are also totally devoid of fruit. Many contain around 300 calories, the amount of calories in one measly bagel. Most frozen entrees are going to be brimming with sodium. (The companies taste-test products with the average American's taste preferences in mind. And the average American likes salt.)

You can add an extra half-cup of noodles or rice, half-cup of steamed or frozen vegetables, and a piece or two of fruit to help round out the entrees (which is what I did when trying the entrees listed on pages 121-122).

Frozen Entrees

	Cal.	Carbs (g)	Fat (g,%*)	Pro. (g)	Fiber (g)	Sod. (mg)
Healthy Choice						
Chicken enchiladas suiza	280	43	6 (19%)	14	5	440
Shrimp & vegetables	270	39	6 (20%)	15	6	580
Herb baked fish	340	54	7 (19%)	16	5	480
Traditional breast of turkey	290	40	4.5 (14%)	22	5	460
Chicken enchilada suprema	300	46	7 (21%)	13	4	560
Lean Cuisine						
Chicken with basil cream sauce	270	35	7 (23%)	16	3	580
Chicken in peanut sauce	290	35	6 (19%)	23	4	590
Baked fish with cheddar shells	270	36	6 (20%)	17	4	540
Fiesta chicken (with black beans, rice, and vegetables)	270	36	5 (17%)	19	4	590
Cheese lasagna with lightly chicken breast scaloppini	290	33	8 (25%)	21	3	590
Shrimp and angel hair pasta	290	55	6 (19%)	10	1	590
3-Bean chili	250	38	6 (22%)	10	9	590
The Budget Gourmet						
Three cheese lasagna	310	34	12 (35%)	15	2	700
Fettucini and meatballs in wine sauce with green beans	270	40	7 (23%)	15	3	560

Frozen Entrees, continued

	Cal.	Carbs (g)	Fat (g, %*)	Pro. (g)	Fiber (g)	Sod. (mg)
Marie Calender's						
Chili and cornbread	540	67	21 (35%)	21	7	2,110
Sweet and sour chicken	570	86	15 (24%)	23	7	700
Beef tips in mushroom sauce	430	39	17 (36%)	25	6	1,620
Turkey with gravy and dressing	500	52	19 (34%)	31	4	2,040
Spaghetti and meat sauce	670	85	25 (34%)	31	9	1,160
Cheese ravioli in marinara sauce (with garlic bread)	750	96	29 (35%)	25	1	1,070
Stuffed pasta trio	640	40	18 (25%)	15	5	950
Swanson						
Mexican style combination	470	59	18 (34%)	18	5	1,610
Chicken parmigiana	370	40	17 (41%)	13	4	1,010
Herb roasted chicken breast tenders with rice & vegetables	310	4	7 (20%)	16	3	780
Turkey dinner	310	40	8.5 (25%)	22	5	890

*Percent calories from fat
Saturated fat for all above-mentioned items is between 1 and 9 mg.

But this is defeating the purpose of a frozen entree, now isn't it? I've listed the nutritional information for the following frozen entrees that I found interesting in my supermarket.

Some people with Type II diabetes fare better with a little more fat in their meal (preferably monounsaturated fat). So, I included any non "light" entree that seemed workable.

Frozen pizza

I always have a frozen pizza in my freezer for those dinner emergencies that come up every now and then. There are actually a couple of brands out there that aren't too bad on the taste buds nor on the nutritional scale either. Sometimes the serving size on frozen pizza can be a bit optimistic—so make sure you know what that is if you are doing any nutrition calculations. Here are a couple of my favorites:

DiGiorno Four Cheese Pizza, one-third of a 12-ounce pizza contains: 280 calories, 34 grams carbohydrate, 9 grams fat (29 percent calories from fat), 5 grams saturated fat, 15 grams protein, 20 milligrams cholesterol, 2 grams fiber, and 700 milligrams sodium.

Wolfgang Puck's Mushroom & Spinach Pizza: one-half of a 10.5-ounce pizza contains: 270 calories, 36 grams carbohydrate, 8 grams fat (27 percent calories from fat), 3 grams saturated fat, 14 grams protein, 10 milligrams cholesterol, 5 grams fiber, and 380 milligrams sodium.

Wolfgang Puck's Four Cheese Pizza: one-half of a 9.25-ounce pizza contains: 360 calories, 40 grams carbohydrate, 15 grams fat (37 percent calories from fat), 6 grams saturated fat, 17 grams protein, 25 milligrams cholesterol, 5 grams fiber, and 530 milligrams sodium.

OreIda Bagel Bites Three Cheese: a four-piece serving contains: 190 calories, 25 grams carbohydrate, 6 grams fat (28 percent calories from fat), 3.5 grams saturated fat, 9 grams protein, 15 milligrams cholesterol, 1 gram fiber, and 530 milligrams sodium.

OreIda Bagel Bites Cheese & Pepperoni: a four-piece serving contains: 200 calories, 26 grams carbohydrate, 7 grams fat (32 percent calories from fat), 3.5 grams saturated fat, 9 grams protein, 15 milligrams cholesterol, 1 gram fiber, and 610 milligrams sodium.

Lean Pockets (Reduced Fat) Pepperoni Pizza Deluxe: one pocket contains: 270 calories, 37 grams carbohydrate, 7 grams fat (23 percent calories from fat), 2.5 grams saturated fat, 15 grams protein, 35 milligrams cholesterol, 3 grams fiber, and 580 milligrams sodium.

Frozen desserts

I'm one of those people who, if given a nudge or two, could eat ice cream every day. People become addicted to this wonderful multi-season treat with its cold and creamy feeling. It comes in fun flavors and tops a meal like no other. Ice cream needs at least *some* fat and sugar or it wouldn't be "ice cream." The choices on page 125 are some of the best-tasting "light" options. I included the nutrition information for some of the better sounding sugar-free frozen dessert options—but I can't vouch for the flavor. By the way, in case you are curious, a half-cup of a "light" ice cream contains about 20 milligrams cholesterol. (We don't include cholesterol in the tables because there are so many other items to list. And, for most people, grams of fat and saturated fat have a greater impact on blood lipids.)

Dairy products

We need milk to keep our cereal company, help liquefy our pancake batter or lighten our coffee. The great thing about milk is that you can take out some of the fat and saturated fat and still have milk that does all the things you want it to do. And as you remove the fat, the cholesterol goes, too. For example:

Frozen Deserts

	Calories	Carbs.	Fat (%*)
Ice cream			
Dreyer's Grand Light (Edy's Grand Light):			
Rocky Road	120	17	4 (30%)
Mocha Almond Fudge	120	16	5 (37%)
Mint Chocolate Chip	120	17	4 (30%)
Coffee Mousse Crunch	120	18	4 (30%)
French Silk	120	19	4 (30%)
Dreyers (Edy's) No Sugar Added:			
Fat Free Chocolate Fudge	100	21	0 (0%)
Butter Pecan	110	12	5 (41%)
Vanilla	80	11	3 (34%)
Ice cream Bars: (1 bar)			
Starbucks Frappuccino	110	20	2 (16%)
Nes Quik Ice Screamers	100	11	5 (45%)
Tropicana Orange Cream	70	14	1 (13%)
Tropicana Strawberry 'n Cream	70	14	1.5 (19%)
Eskimo Pie Reduced Fat/No Sugar Added—Dark Chocolate Coating	120	13	8 (60%)
Eskimo Pie Reduced Fat/No Sugar Added—Crisp Rice	120	13	8 (60%)
Other:			
Sara Lee Reduced Fat Pound Cake (quarter cake)	280	42	11 (35%)
Weight Watchers Smart Ones: (1 serving)			
New York Style Cheesecake	150	21	5 (30%)
Chocolate Eclair	150	25	4 (24%)

*Percent calories from fat

Most of the above-mentioned items contain per serving about 3 g protein, between 1 and 3 g saturated fat, and about 50 mg sodium, except for the Eskimo Pie (about 6 g sodium) and the Weight Watchers Smart Ones (about 150 mg).

- Milk goes from 35 mg cholesterol in a cup of whole milk down to 15 mg in a cup of 1% of low-fat.

- Cottage cheese goes from 25 mg cholesterol in a half- cup of small curd cottage cheese down to 10 mg in low-fat.

Dairy Products

	Cal.	Carbs (g)	Fat (g, %*)	Pro. (g)	Sat. (g)	Sod. (mg)
Milk (1 cup)						
Skim milk	90	13	0	9	0	130
Low-fat milk (1%)	120	14	2.5	11	1.5	160
Low-fat milk (2%)	130	13	5	10	3	140
Whole milk	150	13	8	8	5	125
Cottage cheese (1/2 cup)						
Low-fat cottage cheese	80	3	2 (22%)	13	1	340
Small curd	120	4	5 (38%)	14	3	410
Yogurt						
"Light" fat free flavored yogurts (6 ounces)	90	15	0	5	0	75
99% fat-free flavored yogurts (6 ounces)	170	33	2	5	1	80
Lowfat custard style flavored yogurt (6 ounces)	190	32	3	8	2	100

*Percent calories from fat

It gets a little tricky with other dairy products. If you take more than half the fat out of cheese, for example, if you start going past the halfway mark, it starts looking and tasting a lot less like cheese and a lot more like plastic.

No matter what the amount fat, most dairy products should be consumed in reasonable amounts—they all need to be counted into your daily totals because many contribute carbohydrate grams galore (like fat-free flavored yogurts). Then, the other dairy products that are low in carbohydrates need to be counted because they are most likely contributing some fat grams (like cheese). Either way, you want to make sure you are counting them in to see how they help balance your meals or snacks and how they affect your blood sugar in certain amounts.

Cereal

	Cal.	Carb. (g)	Fat (g, %*)	Fib. (g)	Sod. (mg)
All-Bran Extra Fiber, 1/2 cup	50	20	1 (18%)	13	120
Fiber One, 1/2 cup	60	24	1 (15%)	13	130
All-Bran original, 1/2 cup	80	24	1 (11%)	10	65
100% Bran, 1/3 cup	80	22	.5 (6%)	8	120
Kellogg's Raisin Bran	200	47	1.5 (7%)	8	370
Post Raisin Bran	190	47	1 (5%)	8	300
Shredded Wheat 'n Bran, 1 1/4 cup	200	47	1 (4%)	8	0
Bite Size Frosted Mini-Wheats	200	48	1 (5%)	6	5
Cracklin Oat Bran, 3/4 cup	190	35	7 (33%)	6	170
Raisin Bran Crunch, 1 1/4 cup	210	50	1 (4%)	5	250
Total Raisin Bran	180	43	1 (5%)	5	240
Bran Flakes, 3/4 cup	100	24	.5 (4%)	5	220
Complete Wheat Bran Flakes, 3/4 cup	90	23	.5 (9%)	5	220
Crunchy Corn Bran, 3/4 cup	90	23	1 (10%)	5	250
Spoon Size Shredded Wheat	170	41	.5 (26%)	5	0
Mini-Wheats (Raisin), 3/4 cup	180	42	1 (5%)	5	5
Frosted Shredded Wheat	190	44	1 (5%)	5	10
100% Whole Grain Wheat Chex	180	41	1.5 (8%)	5	420
Fruit & Fibre (Dates, Raisins, and Walnuts)	210	42	3 (13%)	5	280
Grape Nuts, 1/2 cup	210	47	1 (4%)	5	350
Raisin Nut Bran, 3/4 cup	200	41	4 (18%)	5	250
Crisp-Raisin Oatmeal	210	45	2 (8%)	4	220
Banana Nut Crunch (Post)	250	43	6 (22%)	4	250

*Percent calories from fat

Cereal

Whether you prefer it hot, cold, wet, or dry, most of us like some type of cereal. If you eat cereal at least three times a week, that means you sit down to a bowl of cereal about 156 times a year. So, which cereals you choose to eat can make a big difference in, for one thing, the amount of fiber you get.

Most cereals, these days are relatively low in fat, which is actually good because most cereal manufacturers use the partially hydrogenated type of vegetable oils. What distinguishes one cereal from another is usually its sugar and fiber content. I've listed the cereals with 4 grams or more fiber per serving, starting with the highest fiber cereals. The grams of carbohydrate for each are also listed in the table.

Many of you will probably do better with cereal as breakfast or as a snack, if you add some fat to this mostly carbohydrate meal. Low-fat milk is a pretty good way to do this. (I've listed some milk in the table below so you can count it in with your cereal totals.) If you have room left in your carbohydrate breakfast budget, you can top your cereal with sliced banana or berries!

If you're wondering where the Cheerios and whole grain Wheaties are...

They contain 3 grams of fiber per serving so they didn't quite make the list.

Crackers and cookies

Most manufacturers use hydrogenated vegetable oils to make their crackers and cookies. Which means most of these products contribute those undesirable trans fatty acids. Until companies start using liquid canola oil to make their products, the only way to eat crackers and cookies that contain fewer trans fatty acids, then, is to choose crackers and cookies that are lower in fat overall. Look for the reduced fat varieties of either—many taste terrific.

Remember, you aren't supposed to eat half the box. Stick to a "serving" at a time. The amount of cookies and cracker per serving is listed on the box. In order to do this

Cookies

	Cal.	Carbs. (g)	Fat (g, %*)
SnackWell's Double Chocolate Chip cookies, 13	130	22	3 (21%)
SnackWell's Mint Creme, 2	110	19	3.5 (29%)
SnackWell's Creme Sandwich cookies, 2	110	20	3 (25%)
Nabisco Reduced Fat Chips Ahoy! cookies, 3	140	22	5 (32%)
Nabisco Teddy Grahams Chocolatey Chip cookies, 24	130	23	4.5 (31%)
Pepperidge Farm Reduced Fat Oatmeal cookies, 1	100	18	3 (27%)

*Percent calories from fat
The above-mentioned cookies contain 1 to 2 g protein, less than or equal to 1 g fiber, about 1 g saturated fat, and 150 sodium per serving.

though, the crackers and cookies have to taste great and satisfy even the most hard-to-please palates. I've listed what I consider the better-tasting reduced-fat cookies in the table above.

Convenient spaghetti sauces

In order to be included in the list of store-bought sauces that follow, the sauce *had* to contain canola or olive oil (high monounsaturated fat oils). If you've tasted some of the bottled sauces before, I fully realize you may be rather skeptical about buying prepared sauces. This is different.

The following marinara/spaghetti sauces are the only ones that sit on the shelf at room temperature—and they are really pretty good. You can always add in your own super-lean ground beef, mushrooms, garlic, onion, and other spices if you want to dress them up a little. The rest

Pasta Sauces

	Cal.	Carbs. (g)	Fat
Red Sauces (1/2 cup)			
Five Brothers			
Grilled Eggplant & Parmesan	100	13	3
Grilled Summer Vegetable	80	11	3
Mushroom & Garlic Grill	90	12	3
Marinara w/ Burgundy Wine	90	11	3
Classico			
Tomato & Basil	50	9	1
Fire-Roasted Tomato & Garlic	60	10	1
Sutter Home			
Italian Style w/ fresh onions and herbs	80	12	2
Basilla			
Roasted Garlic & Onion	80	12	3.5
Mushroom & Garlic	70	11	2
Tomato & Basil	70	12	1.5
Marinara	70	11	2
Pesto (1/4 cup)			
Contadino Reduced Fat Pesto with Basil	230	111	8
Safeway Select Verdi Classic Pesto	240	72	2
Light Alfredo Sauce (1/4 cup)			
Contadina	80	5	5
Safeway Select Verdi	80	5	5

Most of the red sauces mentioned here contain 0.5 g or less saturated fat, 2 to 3 g protein, 2 to 3 g fiber, and between 390 and 610 mg sodium per serving. Most of the Pesto or Alfredo sauces contain 3 to 4 g protein, between 5 and 20 mg cholesterol, and about 500 mg or less sodium per serving.

of the sauces can be found either in the frozen food section (next to the frozen raviolis) or in the refrigerated "fresh pasta" section.

For bottled spaghetti sauce (normally low in fat and high in carbohydrate), I've listed the brands that contain some olive or canola oil, which means they will contribute some monounsaturated fat. Some people may have

High Monounsaturated Fat Salad Dressings and Spreads

	Cal.	Carbs. (g)	Fat (g)
Mayonnaise: 1 tablespoon*			
Safeway Select Real Mayonnaise w/canola	100	0	11
Spectrum Canola Mayo	100	0	12
Spectrum Lite Canola Eggless Mayonnaise	35	1	3
Salad dressing: 2 tablespoons**			
Kraft Special Collection			
Sun Dried Tomato	60	4	4.5
Italian Pesto	70	5	5.5
Balsamic Vinaigrette	110	1	12
Kraft—Light Done Right			
Red Wine Vinaigrette	50	3	4.5
Italian	50	2	4.5
Raspberry Vinaigrette	60	6	4
Cucumber Ranch	60	2	5.5
Catalina	80	9	5
Kraft			
Roasted Garlic Vinaigrette	50	3	4.5
Caesar Parmesan	60	1	5
Newman's Own			
Dynamite Lite Italian	45	3	4
Balsamic Vinaigrette	90	3	9

*Mayonnaise: 80 or less mg sodium and 1 g saturated fat per serving
**Salad dressing: Between 230 and 480 mg sodium and 1 g saturated fat per serving

better post-pasta blood sugars if there is some fat in there somewhere. Obviously, if you've found one you like that is fat-free, go for it.

High monounsaturated fat salad dressings and spreads

The products on the following page contain exclusively the high monounsaturated fat vegetable oils: canola oil, olive oil, or a combination of the two.

Sugar products

Last but not least, here are a handful of sugar-free or reduced-sugar products that might help you cut down on some extra calories from carbohydrate.

Canned fruits in lightly sweetened juice offer canned fruits year round with less sugar than regular canned fruits.

A half-cup peaches canned in lightly sweetened peach juices contain 80 calories, 19 grams carbohydrate, 1-gram protein, 1-gram fiber, and 20 milligrams sodium.

A half-cup apricot halves in lightly sweetened juice contains 60 calories, 16 grams carbohydrate, 0 gram fat, 0 gram protein, 1 gram fiber, and 10 milligrams sodium.

Jell-O Sugar Free Instant Pudding is available in several flavors. One serving of chocolate flavor contains 35 calories, 8 grams carbohydrate, 0-gram fat, <1-gram protein, <1-gram fiber, and 320 milligrams sodium.

Jell-O Sugar Free Gelatin Desserts are available in several flavors. Use them in your favorite Jell-O recipes or as a quick, low-calorie snack.

Reduced calorie pancake syrups can be found in regular and butter flavored. One-quarter cup contains about 100 calories, 25 grams carbohydrate, and 130 milligrams sodium.

Low Sugar and Lite Jelly and Preserves come in all sorts of brands and flavors. Smucker's makes low sugar jellies and preserves. A tablespoon contains 25 calories and 6 grams of carbohydrate.

Knott's Berry Farm makes light preserves. A tablespoon contains 20 calories and 5 grams of carbohydrate.

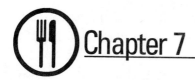 Chapter 7

Restaurant Rules to Eat By

Most people go to restaurants and try to steer clear of one thing—overtly high-fat, high-calorie menu selections. But people with diabetes often have a few more things to worry about when approaching the menu. You need to get a feel for how many carbohydrate grams you might be eating and whether or not it is something that tends to keep your after-meal blood sugars high or not. You might want to choose something that contributes a moderate amount of monounsaturated fat because many find this helps with blood sugar control. You might also be trying to keep saturated fat and trans fatty acids low and omega-3 fatty acids (found in fish and some plant foods) high, to help protect your heart. Many of you may also need to count protein and potassium if you are on dialysis.

That's quite a bit to have on your plate (so to speak). All this could very well take the fun out of eating out, couldn't it? The trick is finding the happy medium between counting what you need to count and ordering and enjoying foods you like. It can be done. It just takes a little practice. Knowing the grams of fat, fiber, and carbohydrate for various menu selections helps too.

Cutting fat and calories when eating out

Remember some people with diabetes control their blood sugar better if they aren't on a very low-fat diet but are on a moderate fat diet (around 30 to 35 percent calories from fat). If you are in this group it is particularly important that you choose monounsaturated fats and omega-3 and omega-9 fatty acids (olive oil, canola oil, fish) whenever possible. No matter which group you are in, though, you will want to avoid "high" animal fat foods which quickly load on extra calories and saturated fat. One of the downfalls of eating out is the hefty portions of meat/dairy you are often served. There are a few things you can do to keep this in check:

- The lean cuts of beef at restaurants are usually filet mignon, sirloin, sirloin tips, or chopped sirloin while the fatter cuts are rib eye, prime rib, porterhouse, and T-bone.

- Make sure your "meat" dish is accompanied by lots of vegetables (beans when possible). The vegetables will help fill you up so you won't be tempted to overdo the meat, and the vegetables and beans help boost fiber totals, too (good for your health and your blood sugars).

- Order the quarter-pounder instead of the one-third pound or half-pound hamburger and load up on lettuce, tomato, catsup and mustard, instead of mayonnaise, "special sauces," and cheese.

- Order the "petite" or "junior" portions of meat, prime rib, and steaks when available.

- Automatically cut your steak, pork chop, ham, or roasted chicken in half and take the rest home for tomorrow's sandwich.

- Ask the restaurant to make your "three-egg" omelet with Egg Beaters egg substitute or one egg blended with three egg whites.

- Avoid extra cheese, and try to keep your servings of heavy cheese dishes (pizza, cheese enchiladas, lasagna, etc.) moderate.

To avoid excessive calories in general, you basically need to avoid ordering foods made with *lots* of:

- Butter or margarine: each tablespoon of butter contains 11.5 grams fat and 102 calories.

- Mayonnaise: each tablespoon of mayonnaise contains 11 grams of fat and 100 calories. (Creamy mayonnaise-based salad dressings are dripping with fat grams. Remember one restaurant ladle adds up to two tablespoons of dressing worth around 25 grams of fat.)

- Cream: one-quarter cup of liquid whipping cream contains 22 grams fat and 205 calories.

- Oil: each tablespoon of oil contains 14 grams fat and 120 calories. Avoid deep fried anything, even if it is something healthful, such as chicken or seafood. Have it grilled instead.

- Sugar: it is loaded with calories. Not that you can't have any, but it helps to split the dessert with someone at the table or eat half and bring the other half home.

Restaurant chain menu picks

Steakhouse chains

There are many steakhouse chains across the country and most of them do *not* provide any nutrition information for their interested patrons (shame on them). Hopefully it's obvious that you should avoid the gigantic, battered, and deep fried onion which, rumor has it, contains more than 100 grams of fat. Sampling, however, is manageable as long as it adds up to a few savored bites.

Even if you avoid everything that is deep fried (not just because of the fat and calories but because anything deep fried seems to cause high blood sugars for many people), what about the other items? If you want to have steak, which is best for you? There are few things that, no matter which steakhouse you're in, will help put you in the nutritional driver's seat:

- Ask that the chef cook your meat without butter or added fat.
- Order your meat in small portions or have the kitchen cut a large portion in half and put the second half immediately into a doggy bag.
- Order your baked potato with butter and sour cream on the side.
- Order your salad with the dressing on the side.
- Trim the visible chunks of fat from your steak.

I did some investigating and came up with the nutrition information for some typical steakhouse menu items. The actual nutrition content of your particular steakhouse item might be higher in fat and calories but the table on the next page will get you in the ballpark. Sodium content varies greatly from restaurant to restaurant.

Menu Items: Steakhouses

	Carbs. (g)	Fat (g [%*])	Pro. (g)	Fib. (g)	Cals.
Entrées					
Grilled chicken	1	2 (15%)	25	n/a	120
Grilled chicken sandwich	39	4 (11%)	33	n/a	324
Grilled salmon (4 oz.)	1	10 (42%)	34	n/a	240
Sirloin tips w/ pepper & onions	4	8 (35%)	27	n/a	203
Spicy BBQ chicken Sandwich	45	5 (12%)	34	n/a	368
Homestyle chicken Fillet	21	9 (37%)	13	n/a	217
Junior sirloin steak	0	10 (46%)	25	n/a	194
Filet mignon, 1 (5.5 oz. cooked)	0	15 (44%)	44	0	330
Smothered steak sandwich	36	15 (31%)	34	n/a	430
Sirloin steak	0	16 (51%)	34	n/a	285
Country steak with gravy	44	25 (42%)	32	n/a	530
Sides					
Baked potato, plain	31	0	3	3	130
Broccoli spears	5	0	3	3	35
Corn, 4 oz.	28	1.5 (9%)	4	3	120
BBQ beans (4 oz.)	25	2 (14%)	6	5	150
Rice pilaf (1/2 cup)	23	3.5 (23%)	2	.5	135
Dinner roll, 1	14	2 (22%)	2	1	85
Cornbread, 1 pc.	28	5 (26%)	4.5	1.5	175
Cinnamon apples	34	5 (26%)	0	2	172
Mashed potatoes,.5 cup	18	5 (35%)	2	2	115
Biscuit, 1	29	15 (50%)	5	1	270
Soups (1 cup)					
Vegetable beef	18	2 (15%)	7	3	120
Clam chowder, New England	17	9 (45%)	3	1.5	180
Chili w/ beans	25	9 (30%)	23	5	270

*Percent calories from fat

Menu Items: Chili's (Guiltless Grill)

	Carbs. (g)	Fat (g [%*])	Fib. (g)	Cal.
Veggie Pasta	98	11 (17%)	16	590
Veggie Pasta with chicken	102	13 (17%)	17	696
Chicken Platter	83	7 (11%)	12	563
Chicken Sandwich	83	7 (12%)	18	527
Chicken Salad with dressing	27	3 (11%)	6	254

*Percent calories from fat

Chili's

Chili's has a "Guiltless Grill" section in their menu featuring about five lower-fat entrées ranging from 3 grams fat and 254 calories to 13 grams fat and 696 calories. All of these are really high in fiber too. To increase the fat grams a little (to an amount that, for some, encourages a better post-meal blood glucose) you can always have a side salad with some vinagrette dressing. There are many other great choices on the Chili's menu too. The selections above have a good chance of fitting into your diabetic, carbo-counting eating plan.

Denny's

Denny's should be commended for being one of the only restaurant chains that willingly offers nutrition information for every single menu item. I wish there were more restaurant chains like this one. All the nutritional information you need to know is on the next page.

Boston Market

For more information on Boston Market's menu choices, check out the menu selections on page 140.

Menu Items: Denny's

	Carbs. (g)	Fat (g [%*])	Pro. (g)	Fib. (g)	Cal.	Sod. (mg)
Breakfast Menu:						
Oatmeal	18	2 (18%)	5	3	100	175
Grits	18	0 (0%)	2	0	80	520
French Toast without syrup or butter	54	24 (42%)	16	3	507	594
Buttermilk Hotcakes (3) without syrup or butter	95	7 (13%)	12	3	491	1,818
Ham, grilled slice	2	3 (29%)	15	0	94	761
Salads/Sandwiches/Soups						
Grilled chicken Sandwich	52	19 (34%)	34	3	509	1,809
Garden Burger	75	33 (44%)	18	8	665	1,051
Charleston Chicken s/w	53	32 (45%)	35	4	632	1,967
Turkey Breast w/ multigrain	39	26 (49%)	23	5	476	1,107
Garden Chicken Delite Salad	33	6 (18%)	30	6	300	1,300
Chili w/ cheese topping	21	19 (42%)	26	7	401	1,039
Split Pea Soup	18	6 (37%)	8	2	146	819
Dinners						
Pot Roast Dinner w/ gravy (add sides)	6	11 (37%)	40	0	265	1,165
Roast Turkey & Stuffing w/ gravy (add sides)	63	27 (35%)	47	0	701	2,346
Grilled Chicken Breast Dinner (add sides)	0	4 (28%)	24	0	130	566
Grilled Alaskan Salmon Dinner (add sides)	1	4 (17%)	43	0	210	103
Chicken Strips (add sides)	55	25 (35%)	47	0	635	1,510

*Percent calories from fat

Olive Garden

A sample of Olive Garden's health-concious menu choices can be seen on page 141.

Menu Items: Boston Market

	Carbs. (g)	Fat (g [%*])	Pro. (g)	Fib. (g)	Cal. (mg)	Sod.
1/4 White Meat Chicken, no skin	2	4 (21%)	33	0	170	480
5 oz. Skinless Rotisserie Turkey Breast	1	1 (6%)	36	0	170	850
5 oz. (lean) Hearth Honey Ham	9	9 (38%)	30	0	210	1490
Teriyaki Chicken 1/4 white w/ skin	17	12 (32%)	40	0	340	890
Southwest Savory Chicken, 1 portion	26	15 (35%)	40	4	400	1670
Baked Sweet Potato, 1	94	7 (15%)	6	10	460	510
BBQ Baked Beans 3/4 cup	48	5 (17%)	8	12	270	540
Black Beans and Rice, 1 cup	45	10 (30%)	8	5	300	1050
New Potatoes, 3/4 cup	25	2.5 (17%)	3	2	130	150
Red Beans and Rice, 1 cup	45	5 (19%)	8	4	260	1050
Rice Pilaf, 2/3 cup	32	5 (25%)	5	2	180	600
Steamed Vegetables (2/3 cup)	7	.5 (14%)	2	3	35	35
Zucchini Marinara, 3/4 cup	7	3 (41%)	1	2	60	330
Corn Bread, 1 mini loaf	33	6 (25%)	3	1	200	390
Turkey Sandwich, no cheese or sauce	61	3.5 (8%)	45	4	400	1070
Ham Sandwich, no cheese or sauce	66	8 (16%)	25	4	440	1450
Open-faced Turkey Sandwich	61	12 (22%)	37	4	500	2170
BBQ Chicken Sandwich	84	9 (15%)	30	3	540	1690
Chicken Noodle Soup, 1 cup	12	4.5 (31%)	11	2	130	1310
Chicken Chili 1 cup	21	7 (27%)	18	6	220	1000

Menu Items: Olive Garden

	Carbs. (g)	Fat (g [%*])	Pro. (g)	Cal.	Sod. (mg)
Garden Fare lunch entrées					
Capellini Pomodoro	52	11 (28%)	9	340	700
Capellini Primavera	58	7 (19%)	14	350	820
Capellini Primavera w/ chicken	59	13 (23%)	39	510	1,550
Chicken Giardino	40	7 (21%)	20	300	910
Linguine alla Marinara	48	6 (20%)	8	280	510
Penne Arrabbiata	49	7 (22%)	8	300	530
Shrimp Primavera	53	9 (18%)	36	440	830
Garden Fare dinner entrées					
Capellini Pomodoro	84	17 (28%)	16	550	1,090
Capellini Primavera	99	12 (18%)	23	600	1,450
Capellini Primavera with chicken	101	18 (21%)	48	760	2,190
Chicken Giardino	59	8 (16%)	36	460	1,180
Grilled Chicken Capri	45	9 (17%)	58	500	640
Linguine alla Marinara	79	9 (19%)	14	450	770
Penne Arrabbiata	67	11 (23%)	12	410	800
Shrimp Primavera	103	14 (15%)	69	830	1,390
Other:					
Minestrone Soup (6 oz)	18	1 (9%)	5	100	610
Plain Breadstick	26	1.5 (10%)	5	140	270

*Percent calories from fat
Fiber information was not available for these items

Good choices at pizza parlors

Some pizza chains have higher fat pizza crust while others have the more traditional, bread-type crust. Test the fat content of your pizza by laying your slice of pizza on a thick napkin. Do the grease spots form a triangle where the crust was? The grease from the oil is an indication of the fat content. It's best to frequent the pizza places that have the more traditional bread crusts—that's half the battle. Domino's, for example, makes a hand tossed pizza crust and a pan crust. Choose the hand tossed one because it has half the fat and saturated fat of deep dish pizza.

The second factor in choosing the healthier pizza pie is the toppings: the cheese and all the trimmings. If you ask to have the pizza made with less cheese, this will definitely help. I know you feel silly doing this, but many of these restaurants really do put on more cheese than pizza really needs. If you are used to the typical combination pizza (sausage and pepperoni) this next tip could be a tough one. If you top your pizza with items that don't add fat calories, but instead add nutrition and fiber—you are hitting the nutrition jackpot. You see, people usually don't have any vegetables with their pizza meal (unless they order a salad), so why not top your pizza with the vegetables you like and make it a more complete meal? Hopefully you like a couple of the following vegetable toppings: peppers, onions, mushrooms, zucchini, fresh tomatoes, broccoli, artichoke hearts, and topping fruits, such as pineapple. The leaner meat toppings are Canadian bacon and ham.

Blood sugar beware...

Pizza seems to be one of those foods that raises blood sugar higher than you might expect given the amount of carbohydrates. You might find you tolerate your pizza better if you have a side salad, heavy on the kidney beans before you eat your pizza. This is probably not a good time to be eating a big slice of cake either. Try two large-size slices of cheese pizza and see how your blood sugar fares. Two slices will bring you to about 45 grams of carbohydrate.

Menu Items: Blimpie (per 6-inch sub)

	Carbs. (g)	Fat (g [%*])	Pro. (g)	Fib. (g)	Cal.	Sod. (mg)
Blimpie Best	47	13 (28%)	26	4	410	1,480
Ham and Swiss	47	13 (27%)	25	5	430	970
Turkey	51	4.5 (13%)	19	3	320	690
Roast Beef	47	4.5 (12%)	27	2	340	870
Club	53	13 (26%)	30	3	450	1,350
Grilled Chicken	52	9 (20%)	28	2	400	960
Grilled Chicken Salad	13	12 (31%)	47	0	350	1,190

*Percent of calories from fat

Good choices at sandwich shops

There are really great sandwich choices at the following sandwich restaurants. They are good places to go when you have a few minutes and/or a few dollars for lunch. The nutritional facts for the sandwiches are analyzed using white bread. If you opt for the whole or part wheat selections, your grams of fiber might go up about 2 to 4 grams a sandwich.

Unless noted, the following nutritional data does not include cheese and condiments—such as mayonnaise and salad dressing. If you add mayonnaise or salad dressing, you'll need to add this into the equation (see the table above). Good news, though. Subway offers light mayonnaise. Other condiments available upon request are mustard, vinegar, and an olive oil blend.

Good choices at fast food chains

It's just too easy to eat a horrendously high fat, high calorie meal at your average fast food chain. These foods contain the heart damaging types of fat and you'd be hard pressed to find a fruit or vegetable to munch on. Some of the restaurants now offer side salads and fat free or light salad dressing to go with your sandwich selection. If you

Menu Items: Subway

	Carbs. (g)	Fat (g [%*])	Pro (g)	Cal.	Sod. (mg)
Per 6-inch subs					
Veggie Delite	44	3 (11%)	9	237	593
Turkey Breast	46	4 (12%)	18	289	1,403
Turkey Breast & Ham	46	5 (15%)	18	295	1,361
Ham	45	5 (15%)	19	302	1,319
Roast Beef	45	5 (15%)	20	303	939
Subway Club	46	5 (14%)	21	312	1,352
Seafood & Crab (made w/ lite mayo)	45	10 (26%)	20	347	884
Roasted Chicken Breast	47	6 (16%)	27	348	978
Steak & Cheese	47	10 (23%)	30	398	1,117
Subway Melt (includes cheese)	46	12 (28%)	23	382	1,746
Per Deli Style Sandwich (on deli style roll)					
Turkey	38	4 (15%)	12	235	944
Ham	37	4 (15%)	11	234	773
Roast Beef	38	4 (15%)	13	245	638
Tuna (w/ light mayo)	38	9 (29%)	11	279	583
Salads (not including dressing)					
Veggie Delite	10	1 (18%)	2	51	308
Turkey Breast	12	2 (18%)	11	102	1,117
Subway Club	12	3 (21%)	11	126	1,067
Roast Beef	11	3 (23%)	12	117	654
Ham	11	3 (23%)	12	116	1,034
Turkey Breast & Ham	11	3 (25%)	11	109	1,076
Roasted Chicken Breast	13	4 (22%)	20	162	693
Steak & Cheese	13	8 (34%)	22	212	832

*Percent calories from fat

know you will be eating at a fast food restaurant, bring along some fruit and raw vegetables (carrots, celery) to help round off the meal. I know this sounds totally

Menu Items: Jack in the Box

	Carbs. (g)	Fat (g [%*])	Pro. (g)	Fib. (g)	Cal.	Sod. (mg)
Chicken Teriyaki Bowl	128	4 (5%)	26	3	670	1730
Pancakes with Bacon	59	9 (22%)	12	3	370	1020
Chicken Fajita Pita	25	9 (29%)	24	3	280	840
Breakfast Jack	30	12 (39%)	17	1	280	920
Hamburger	30	12 (38%)	12	2	280	560
Hamburger with Cheese	30	16 (45%)	14	2	320	760
Chicken Breast Pieces (5)	24	17 (42%)	27	1	360	970
Garden Chicken Salad	8	9 (40%)	23	3	200	420
Side Salad	3	3 (54%)	2	3	50	75
Low Calorie Italian Dressing (4 tbsp)	2	1.5 (54%)	0	0	25	670

*Percent calories from fat

Menu Items: Kentucky Fried Chicken

	Carbs. (g)	Fat (g [%*])	Pro. (g)	Fib. (mg)	Cal. (mg)	Sod. (mg)
Tender Roast Chicken Breast w/out skin	1	4.3 (23%)	31.4	0	169	797
Tender Roast Chicken Thigh w/o skin	<1	5.5 (46%)	13	0	106	312
BBQ Flavored Chicken sandwich	28	8 (28%)	17	2	256	782
BBQ Baked Beans	33	3 (14%)	6	6	190	760
Corn on the Cob	35	1.5 (9%)	5	2	150	20
Green Beans	7	1.5 (30%)	1	3	45	730
Mean Greens	11	3 (38%)	4	5	70	650

*Percent calories from fat

Menu Items: McDonald's

	Carbs. (g)	Fat (g [%*])	Pro. (g)	Fib. (g)	Cal.	Sod. (mg)
Hamburger	34	9 (31%)	13	2	250	580
Cheeseburger	35	13 (37%)	15	2	320	820
Grilled Chicken Deluxe	38	20 (41%)	27	4	440	1040
Grilled Chicken Deluxe (no mayo)	38	5 (15%)	27	4	300	930
Grilled Chicken Salad Deluxe w/ 1 pkg. fat-free Herb dressing	18	1.5 (8%)	21	3	170	570
Grilled Chicken Salad w/ 1/2 pkg. Caesar Dressing	10.5	8.5 (38%)	22	3	200	465
Egg McMuffin	27	12 (38%)	17	1	290	790
Hotcakes (plain)	58	9 (23%)	9	2	340	540
Hotcakes w/ 2 pats margarine & syrup**	104	18 (26%)	9	2	610	600
Lowfat Apple Bran Muffin	61	3 (10%)	6	3	300	380
Vanilla Reduced Fat Ice Cream Cone	23	4.5 (27%)	4	0	150	75
Small Shake (all flavors)	60	9 (22%)	11	0	360	180

*Percent calories from fat

**The carbohydrate and calorie count would reduce if only 1/2 syrup packet was used.

impractical, but if you eat fast food often, this is an important habit to get into.

When it comes to burgers, bigger is not better. The smaller the hamburger, the lower the percent of calories from fat. Some of this has to do with the fact that smaller hamburgers have more bun per square inch of burger. But some of it is because the bigger burgers get the fancier (and higher fat) sauces while the small burgers are served with catsup and mustard. Each fast food chain has its pluses and minuses. Take a look at the list that follows to find some selections you might enjoy.

Menu Items: Wendy's

	Carbs. (g)	Fat (g [%++])	Pro. (g)	Fib. (g)	Cal.	Sod. (mg)
Sandwiches						
Grilled Chicken	35	8 (23%)	27	2	310	790
Jr. Hamburger	34	10 (33%)	15	2	270	610
Jr. Cheeseburger	34	13 (36%)	17	2	320	830
+Spicy Chicken	43	15 (33%)	28	2	410	1,280
Plain Single	31	16 (40%)	24	2	360	580
+Breaded Chicken	44	18 (37%)	28	2	440	840
Pitas*						
Garden Veggie	52	17 (38%)	11	5	400	760
Chicken Caesar	48	18 (33%)	34	4	490	1,320
Garden Ranch Chicken	51	18 (34%)	30	5	480	1,180
Per salad**						
Side Salad	5	3 (45%)	4	2	60	180
Caesar Side Salad	7	5 (41%)	10	1	110	650
Deluxe Garden	9	6 (49%)	7	3	110	350
Grilled Chicken	9	8 (36%)	25	3	200	720
Dressing (2 tablespoons)						
Italian, reduced fat	2	3			40	340
Ranch, reduced fat	2	5			60	240
French, fat-free	8	0			35	150
Other						
Sour Cream & Chives Potato	74	6 (14%)	8	8	380	40
Broccoli & Cheese Potato	80	14 (27%)	9	9	470	470
Chili, small serving	2	17 (30%)	15	5	210	800

*The pitas are made with reduced-fat Caesar vinaigrette (70 calories, 7 grams fat per tablespoon) or a reduced-fat garden ranch sauce (50 calories, 4.5 grams fat per tablespoon).

**The salad values below do not include salad dressing. Add in the nutrition info for the salad dressing of your choice.

+Order these sandwiches with ketchup or reduced calorie honey mustard instead of the mayonnaise and you'll reduce the sandwich totals by about 3 grams fat for ketchup and 1.5 grams fat for the honey mustard.

++Percent calories from fat

Menu Items: Burger King

	Carbs. (g)	Fat (g [%*])	Pro. (g)	Fib. (g)	Cal.	Sod. (mg)
Whopper Jr. (without mayo)	28	15 (44%)	19	2	320	530
Hamburger	27	15 (44%)	19	1	320	520
BK Big Fish sandwich (no tartar sauce)	59	14 (27%)	23	3	460	850
BK Broiler Chicken sandwich (nomayo)	45	9 (22%)	29	2	370	1,060
Chicken sandwich (without mayo)	54	20 (36%)	26	2	500	1,400
Chick'N Crisp (without mayo)	37	16 (39%)	16	3	360	890
Small Vanilla Shake	56	7 (19%)	10	1	330	250
Small French Fries	32	13 (32%)	2	2	250	550

*Percent calories from fat

Bagel shop

I love fresh bagels! Spread with light cream cheese, they are one of my favorite breakfasts. Bagels look innocent enough but they can be trouble for some people with diabetes. There's something about those 40-ish grams of carbohydrates that seems to make normal blood sugars difficult first thing in the morning for many people with Type II diabetes. But there are a few things you can do to improve your post-bagel blood sugars.

Try whole grain bagels or oat bran bagels to see if that makes a difference. Make sure you balance your mostly carbohydrate bagel with some protein and a little fat. You can do this by spreading your bagel with light cream cheese or filling a savory bagel with some reduced-fat cheese and a slice of lean ham.

Menu Items: Donut Shop

	Carbs. (g)	Fat (g [%*])	Pro. (g)	Fib. (g)	Cal.	Sod. (mg)
French Cruller	24	7.5 (40%)	1	2	170	140
Cake Donut, Glazed	23	10 (47%)	3	2	192	180
Cinnamon Bun	31	10 (39%)	4	6	220	190
Jelly Donut	25	12 (48%)	4	3	221	190
Croissant	26	12 (47%)	5	7	231	424
Yeast Donut	26	14 (50%)	4	3	242	205
Fruit Danish	45	16 (42%)	5	3	335	333
Cheese Danish	29	25 (62%)	6	5	350	319

*Percent calories from fat

Donut /coffee shop chain

Here is the nutritional information from a national donut/coffee shop chain. We all find ourselves in these places every now and then and we all probably crave donuts every once in a while. When we do—here is some of the nutrition information that can help you make your choices.

Ⓨ¶ Conclusion

ou've heard the expression, you can lead a horse to water but you can't make him drink? I have been dragging my Type II father (whom I love with all my heart) to the water for 15 years, and..well, he's not drinking. Oh sure, every now and then he might sip the water a little, or dip his big toe in. But when it comes right down to it, he's not drinking. He just hasn't been interested in controlling his blood sugars and he has definitely never been willing to find an eating plan that will help his blood sugars. He won't write down what he is eating and the resultant blood sugars so that we can figure out patterns.

For fifteen years I have watched him slowly lose his ability to drive, walk, travel. We are at the point where every other month he is in the hospital for congestive heart or leg infections. Even now he isn't interested in controlling his blood sugars. All I can do now is just love him, keep him company when my mom is working a long day, scratch his back (one of his favorite things), and just generally savor every precious moment my children and I get to spend with him.

I applaud you for being motivated enough to improve your health and diabetes that you finished this book. I can't say I know exactly what you are going through because I don't personally have Type II diabetes...yet. But I do understand. And if this book has somehow made your life with diabetes more enjoyable and more comfortable, than all the long hours of writing and research was well worth it.

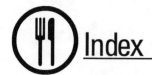 # Index